An Outline of
Ophthalmology

Roger L. Coakes MBBS FRCS DO

Consultant Ophthalmic Surgeon, King's College Hospital, London

Patrick J. Holmes Sellors MA BM BCh FRCS

Surgeon-Oculist to H.M. The Queen;
Consultant Surgeon, Croydon Eye Unit, and the
Royal Marsden Hospital;
Honorary Consultant Surgeon, St George's Hospital, London

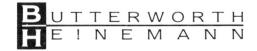

BUTTERWORTH
HEINEMANN

Butterworth-Heinemann Ltd
Linacre House, Jordan Hill, Oxford OX2 8DP

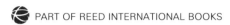 PART OF REED INTERNATIONAL BOOKS

OXFORD   LONDON   BOSTON
MUNICH   NEW DELHI   SINGAPORE   SYDNEY
TOKYO   TORONTO   WELLINGTON

First published 1985
Reprinted 1988, 1990, 1992

© Butterworth-Heinemann Ltd 1988

British Library Cataloguing in Publication Data
Coakes, Roger L.
   An outline of ophthalmology
   1. Eye – diseases and defects
   I. Title   II. Sellors, Patrick, J. Holmes
   617.7   RE46

ISBN 0 7506 0760 2

Printed and bound in Great Britain
by Hartnolls Ltd, Bodmin, Cornwall

To our wives, Mary and Gill

Preface

This outline of ophthalmology has been written for medical students but we hope it will prove to be a useful reference for the various eye problems encountered after qualification.

A symptomatic approach to specific eye disorders has been adopted with a complementary section on ocular involvement in systemic disease. This somewhat arbitrary division has led to repetition in places but we hope that this format will reinforce the point that ophthalmology is not an isolated speciality but an important part of medicine.

We would like to acknowledge the secretarial help of Mrs Eileen Roberts who so ably processed the words of the manuscript. The illustrations are almost entirely the work of Mr Colin Clements and Mr Terry Tarrant to whom we are indebted for their photographic and artistic skills respectively. Additional illustrations of patients were kindly supplied by many of our colleagues and we are particularly grateful to Dr John Dawson, Dr John Anderson, Dr Richard Baker, Dr Nick Evans, Dr Alan Darby, Mr Clive Migdal, Mr Alistair Fielder, Mr Paul Hunter and Mr Geoffrey Davies. Finally, we wish to thank Mr Timothy ffytche and Dr Keith Pettingale for their helpful and constructive criticisms of the text.

Contents

Outline anatomy of the eye

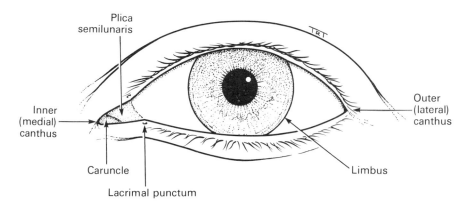

The palpebral aperture.

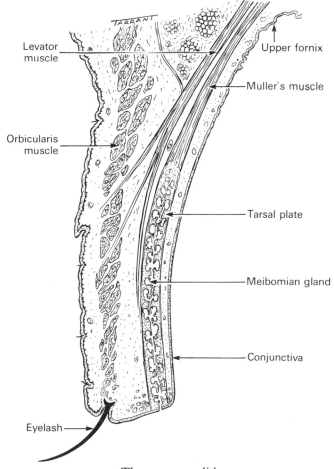

The upper eyelid.

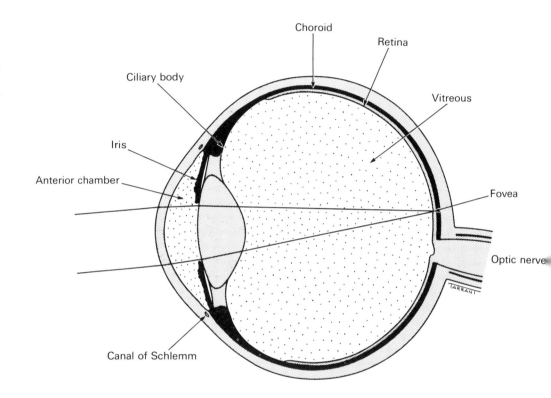

The eye from above.

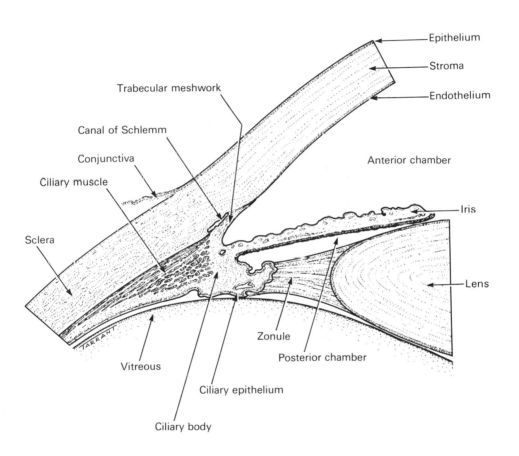

The drainage angle.

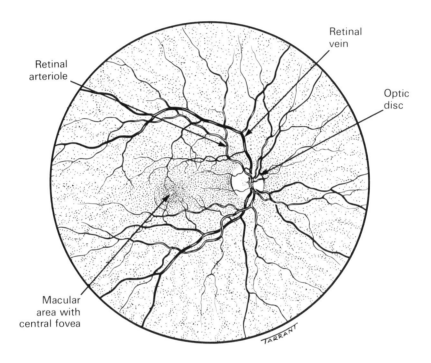

Retinal
vein

Retinal
arteriole

Optic
disc

Macular
area with
central fovea

The ocular fundus.

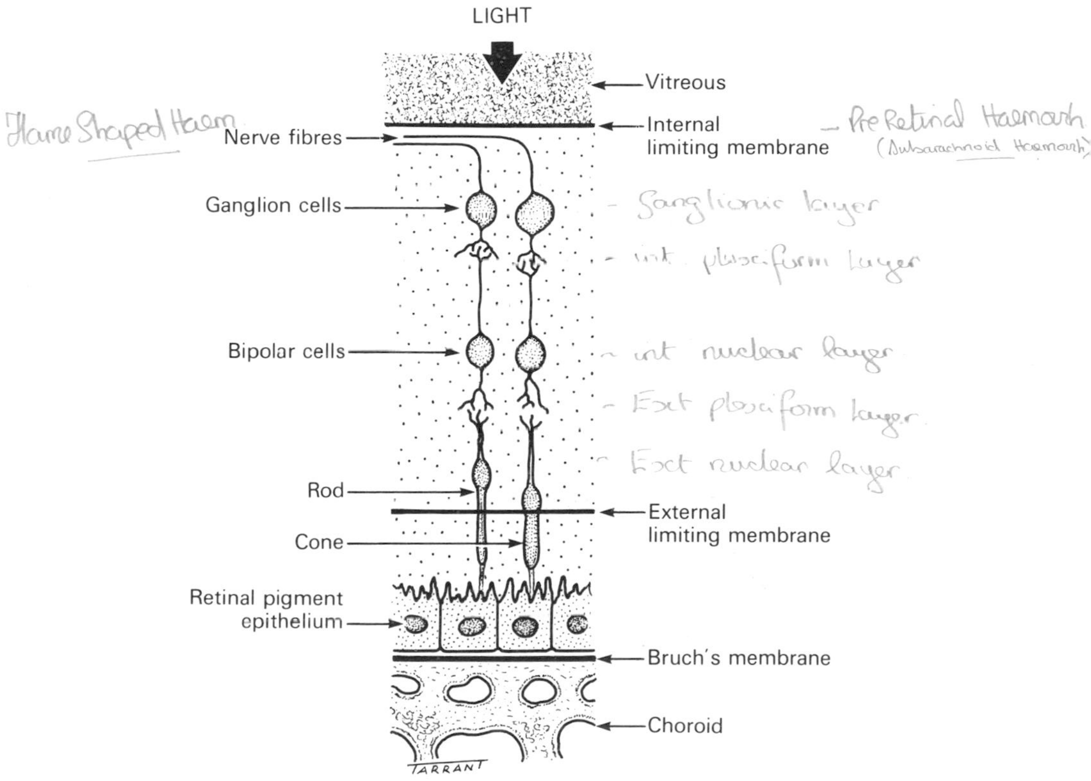
LIGHT
Vitreous
Internal limiting membrane
Nerve fibres
Ganglion cells
Bipolar cells
Rod
Cone
Retinal pigment epithelium
External limiting membrane
Bruch's membrane
Choroid
TARRANT
Flame Shaped Haem
Pre Retinal Haemorrh
(Subarachnoid Haemorrh)
Ganglionic layer
int. plexiform layer
int nuclear layer
Ext plexiform layer
Ext nuclear layer

The retina.

Part 1

Diseases of the eye

Section 1

Loss of vision

Assessment of vision and visual symptoms 1

One of the commonest presenting features in ophthalmology is loss of vision. This may be sudden, gradual or transient and involve either a decline in visual acuity, loss of peripheral field or both. In order to determine the cause it is necessary, in addition to taking a careful history, to be able to assess visual function, interpret visual symptoms and examine the eye with the aid of an ophthalmoscope.

Assessment of visual function

Visual acuity

Visual acuity is a measure of the ability of the eye to discriminate between two points. It is the central vision required for seeing details at all distances.

It is a function of the macular area of the retina, and in particular the central fovea, and is mediated by the retinal cones and their central connections.

Distance vision

The most familiar test of visual acuity is the Snellen chart. This has a series of letters of graduated size, each subtending an angle of 5 minutes of arc at a specific distance. The top letter on the chart subtends this angle at 60 metres while the smallest letters subtend the angle at 5 metres.

The test is conducted at a distance of 6 metres (20 feet) which is optically equivalent to infinity. A patient who can only see the top letter has a visual acuity of 6/60, while a patient who can read down to those letters subtending an angle of 5 minutes of arc at 12 metres has a visual acuity of 6/12. Visual acuity of 6/6 is the accepted normal (in America, expressed as 20/20).

When the visual acuity is less than 6/60 the distance

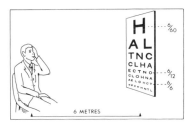

Snellen chart.

13

between the observer and the chart can be reduced (for example 2/60 means that the top letter can only be seen at a distance of 2 metres). Vision below 1/60 can be recorded as the ability to count fingers (CF), to see hand movements (HM) or perceive light (PL). A totally blind eye is unable to perceive light (NPL).

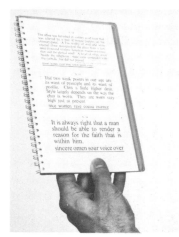

Near vision

Visual acuity at reading distance is measured with varying sizes of printed text. Special books printed in 'Times Roman' type are used. The smallest print is 4.5 or 5.0 point and the largest 48 point. The acuity is prefixed by the letter N (near). N8 is the size of the average newspaper column but normal near vision is N5 or better. N5 is approximately equivalent to 6/12 on the Snellen chart. Books using Jaeger's types are still used. The smallest print, J1, is nearly equivalent to N5.

Near test type.

The measurement of near vision is important as reading is a part of everyday life but it should be used in addition to the Snellen chart and not as an alternative. It is difficult to standardize the test as the text can be held at varying distances from the eyes and the result will also be affected by the degree of illumination.

The Sheridan–Gardiner test

This simple test is designed to measure visual acuity in children below reading age. The child holds a card with seven letters. From a distance of 6 metres the examiner shows the child a single letter (corresponding in size to the Snellen letters) and the child points to the matching letter on his chart. Children as young as two and a half years may be able to manage this test. It is also useful for illiterate patients and for those who do not know Roman letters.

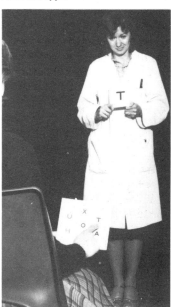

Sheridan–Gardiner test.

Peripheral vision

The field of vision is that portion of space which can be seen by the eye. It is bounded medially by the nose, superiorly by the upper lid or brow and below by the cheek. An area of absent or depressed vision within this field is known as a scotoma. The optic nerve head (optic disc) has no visual receptors and thus results in an absolute scotoma temporal to fixation—*the blind spot*.

The visual field and defects within it can be measured by plotting the light threshold of different

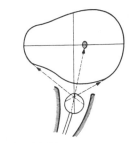

The visual field.

areas of the retina with static lights of varying intensity (static perimetry) or by moving targets of known size and luminance across the field (kinetic perimetry). Accurate charting of the visual fields requires instruments of varying complexity but simple diagnostic assessment is possible with confrontation methods.

A. In each quadrant of the field of vision the patient is asked to state whether one or two fingers are being held up by the examiner.

B. One eye is covered and the patient fixates the examiner's opposite eye. A target, e.g. a neurological pin, is brought in from the periphery and the extent of the patient's visual field, and defects within it, are assessed using the examiner's field as a control.

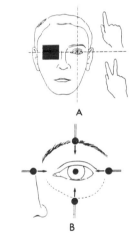

Static perimetry.

   Both of these methods will quickly identify gross field loss such as a homonymous or bitemporal hemianopia. With practise small central and paracentral field defects can be detected by method B.

Colour vision

Normal colour vision is required for certain occupations, for example certain branches of the armed forces and electrical engineering. About 7% of men and 0.5% of women are congenitally colour blind. The defect is usually in red/green differentiation and is hereditary, transmitted as a sex-linked abnormality.

   Colour vision is most easily tested with pseudoisochromatic colour plates such as those of Ishihara and Hardy, Rand & Rittler. Acquired colour defects may be found in macular and optic nerve disease.

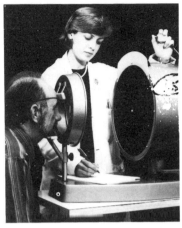

Confrontation methods of testing visual fields.

Refractive errors

By far the commonest cause of defective visual acuity is a refractive error. The cornea and lens focus rays of light onto the retina to form a clear image. A refractive error is present when this focusing cannot be achieved without the aid of a correcting lens.

   The *pinhole test* can indicate whether diminished visual acuity is due to a refractive error. The patient views the Snellen chart through a pinhole made in a card. The small aperture allows only the passage of rays parallel and close to the visual axis which are not

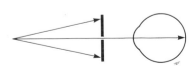

Pinhole effect.

refracted by the cornea and lens. Thus if a lowered acuity improves to normal with the use of a pinhole a refractive error is present.

Emmetropia (the optically normal eye)

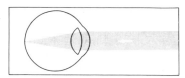
Emmetropia.

Light from infinity is focused onto the retina without accommodation of the lens. Objects nearer than infinity are brought to a focus by accommodation. This is achieved by contraction of the ciliary muscle which slackens the zonule and allows the normal elasticity of the lens to increase its converging power.

Thus, an emmetropic eye does not require any correcting spectacle lens until the power of accommodation is inadequate for reading (*presbyopia*). This leads to the common situation of the middle aged who find that although distance vision remains satisfactory close vision becomes progressively worse, necessitating the wearing of reading glasses.

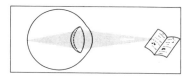
Accommodation.

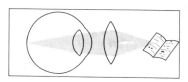
Presbyopia.

Myopia (short sight)

In this state light from infinity is focused in front of the retina producing a blurred image but near objects may be focused satisfactorily without accommodation.

Accommodation increases the converging power of the lens making myopia worse. The reverse process is not possible and myopia can only be corrected by a diverging (concave) lens.

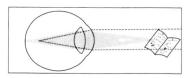
Myopia.

Hypermetropia

In this condition light from infinity is focused behind the retina unless accommodation can correct this. In youth, when the range of accommodation is considerable, the hypermetrope may be able to overcome his refractive error but eventually a converging lens (convex) is required.

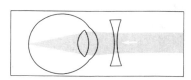
Correction of myopia.

Astigmatism

The major refracting surface of the eye is the cornea. If this is shaped as part of a perfect sphere a point of light will be focused as such on the retina. However, if the corneal surface is aspherical then a point of light is focused as a smudge (astigmatism means 'not a point').

In the majority of cases the maximum and minimum curvatures of the cornea are at right angles to each other (regular astigmatism) and the optical defect can be corrected by the use of cylindrical lenses which

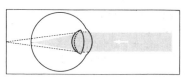
Hypermetropia.

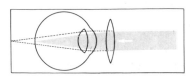
Correction of hypermetropia.

refract light in one axis only. In certain pathological
conditions, e.g. keratoconus and corneal scarring, the
angle between the maximum and minimum curvatures
is less than a right angle (irregular astigmatism) and the
defect can only be corrected with a contact lens or
corneal graft which provide a new spherical refractive
interface.

Visual phenomena

In addition to a decrease in visual acuity, field of vision
or colour discrimination, there are other disturbances
of vision for which the patient may seek advice (double
vision is considered in Chapter 18).

Haloes

Haloes appearing around a point source of light are
caused by diffraction of the light and are corneal or
lenticular in origin.
   Corneal oedema from any cause, but especially from
acutely raised intraocular pressure, results in the
appearance of *rainbow* haloes around white lights.
   Lenticular haloes, caused by early cataract, do not
have a true rainbow appearance and, unlike those due
to an acute rise in intraocular pressure, are seen
whenever a light is looked at.

Floaters

Floating spots in the field of vision are a frequent
complaint. They are always due to opacities in the
vitreous body. The commonest causes are:

Muscae volitantes ('darting flies')
Most individuals experience these fine, almost translucent, particles which dart across the field of vision on
movement of the eye. They are best seen against a plain
background but are most irritating during reading.
They are caused by the remnants of a dense vascular
network which fills the vitreous in fetal life but
regresses before birth. They are of no pathological
significance.

Vitreous detachment
In middle age and beyond the outer cortical vitreous
detaches from the retinal surface as part of a normal
ageing process. A ring of cortical vitreous, previously

previously attached around the optic nerve, casts a shadow on the retina and is frequently described by the patient as a ring or, if broken and irregular, a spider or hairnet.

→ *Blurred Vision*

Vitreous haemorrhage

Extravasation of small amounts of blood into the vitreous may be experienced initially as floating spots but a description of smoke drifting across the sky may be given.

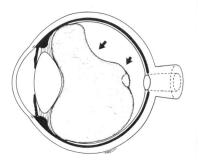

Posterior detachment of the vitreous.

Flashes

This is a common symptom caused by mechanical stimulation of the retinal photoreceptors.

Retinal tear

The combination of flashes and floaters suggest the possibility of a retinal tear which may be the precursor of a retinal detachment.

Retinal traction

Flashes of light also result from retinal traction, most commonly due to vitreous detachment but also occurring as a result of retinal elevation by, for example, a choroidal tumour.

Metamorphopsia

This common symptom takes the form of distortion of central vision or an alteration in image size (macropsia, micropsia) and is almost invariably caused by macular disease.

Patterned and formed images

The typical fortification spectrum of migraine (*see* Chapter 4) is usually diagnostic but is occasionally mistaken for a glaucomatous halo.

Formed hallucinations originate in the temporal and parietal cortex. The commonest causes are epilepsy and drug intoxication.

Examination of the eye that has lost vision

Examination of the pupil reactions and ocular fundus will, in many instances, reveal the cause of loss of vision. An orderly examination of the eye, including the visual field, is important if diagnostic features are not to be missed.

Pupil reactions

Defective reaction of the pupil to light (an _afferent pupillary defect_) in an eye that has lost vision is due to disease of the retina, optic nerve or chiasm. It is never caused by an opacity within the eye, such as a cataract or vitreous haemorrhage nor is it due to disease of the visual pathway posterior to the lateral geniculate body.

Ophthalmoscopy

Red reflex

The red reflex seen with the ophthalmoscope, when held a few inches away from the patient's eye, is due to reflection of light from the choroid. Loss of this red reflex may be total or partial. Absence of the red reflex may be due to dense cataract (gradual loss of vision) or vitreous haemorrhage (sudden loss of vision). Partial loss of the red reflex may be due to cortical lens opacities; a detached retina gives the appearance of a grey reflex.

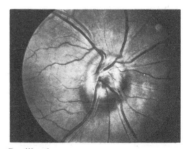
Cortical lens opacities.

Optic disc

Swelling of the optic disc with acute loss of vision suggests local vascular or inflammatory disease of the optic nerve. Papilloedema without loss of vision usually has an intracranial cause.

Pallor of the optic disc may be due to retinal, optic nerve or chiasmal disease.

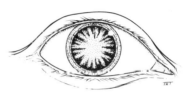
Papilloedema.

Macula

Macular disease is associated with loss of visual acuity and distortion of central vision. It is difficult, and at times, impossible, to assess the macula through the undilated pupil.

Characteristic changes occurring in macular disease include loss of the foveal reflex, pigment disturbance, the presence of refractile bodies and exudative changes.

Retina

1. The retinal vessels. The retinal veins are darker than the retinal arterioles and appear larger in diameter by a

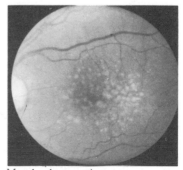
Macular degeneration.

ratio of 3:2. Engorgement of the retinal veins indicates a local circulatory problem associated with slow flow. Attenuation of the retinal arterioles may be due either to occlusive vascular disease or widespread retinal atrophy.

2. Retinal background. Retinal haemorrhages occur in a wide variety of ocular and systemic diseases. Deep retinal haemorrhages are circumscribed while superficial haemorrhages are flame shaped (following the course of the nerve fibres); the distribution of the haemorrhages is frequently of diagnostic value.

True retinal exudates (hard exudates) are due to the accumulation of lipid within the retina from leaking blood vessels. These must be distinguished from 'soft exudates' (cotton-wool spots) which are retinal infarcts.

New vessels arising on the surface of the optic disc or retina are indicative of widespread retinal ischaemia. They do not themselves interfere with vision but bleeding from these fragile vessels does.

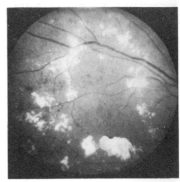

Hard exudates.

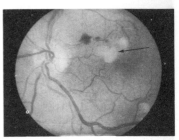

Haemorrhage and retinal infarct (arrowed).

Sudden loss of vision 2

In the *outwardly* normal eye sudden loss of vision is usually caused by disease of the *retina, choroid or optic nerve*.

Diseases and injuries of the anterior part of the eye resulting in sudden loss of vision cause varying degrees of pain and redness and are considered under The Acute Red Eye (Chapter 7) and Trauma (Section V).

Causes of sudden loss of vision

The causes of sudden loss of vision include :

1. **Occlusion of the central retinal vein**
2. **Occlusion of the central retinal artery**
3. **Vitreous haemorrhage**
   - **Retinal detachment**
   - **Optic and retrobulbar neuritis**
   - **Ischaemic optic neuropathy**
   - **Choroiditis**
   - **Homonymous hemianopia**

Sudden loss of vision is a dramatic symptom and is usually *unilateral*. The visual loss is rapid when the cause is vascular but may develop over a period of hours or days if due to inflammation or retinal detachment.

Occlusion of the central retinal vein

Clinical features

The loss of vision is often first noticed on waking. The retinal veins are engorged, tortuous and dark and the optic disc is swollen. Retinal haemorrhages occur along the vessels and extend into the periphery. Retinal infarcts (soft exudates) are common and the posterior retina is oedematous due to impaired venous drainage.

Causes

1. The vein and artery are intimately associated in the optic nerve head and hypertensive and sclerotic changes within the artery contribute to occlusion of the vein.
2. Raised intraocular pressure in chronic glaucoma may compress the central retinal vein at its exit from the eye.
3. Blood disorders causing increased viscosity, e.g. polycythaemia, impede venous flow.

4. Systemic Disorders eg Bechets.

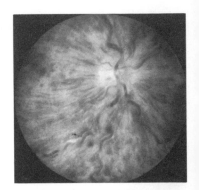

Central retinal vein occlusion.

Management

1. *Mild cases.* If the visual acuity is 6/24 or better the prognosis is good. No treatment is required and the retinal haemorrhages gradually absorb over a period of 2–3 months. Collateral vessels may develop around the optic disc to allow restoration of normal blood flow and may be the only visible sequelae of the vein occlusion.

2. *Severe cases.* The prognosis is poor if the visual acuity is 6/60 or worse. The retinal haemorrhages absorb slowly and the venous drainage of the macular region may be so badly affected as to leave the area chronically oedematous. Widespread retinal ischaemia may result in neovascularization of the iris and drainage angle causing secondary 'thrombotic' glaucoma. This complication can be prevented in photo-coagulation of the retina (*see* Chapter 25). Anticoagulants have no place in the treatment of retinal vein occlusion.

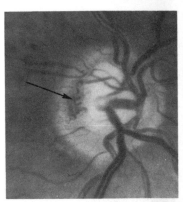

Collateral vessels.

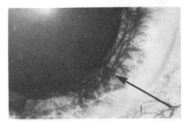

New vessels on iris.

Branch retinal vein occlusion

Frequently occlusions occur at the first major arteriovenous crossing from the optic disc. The haemorrhages are then restricted to the area of retina drained by the vein and visual loss is related to the degree of macular involvement.

A branch retinal vein occlusion is nearly always an indication of generalized vascular disease. Treatment is seldom required though photocoagulation may be necessary if retinal neovascularization occurs. The development of thrombotic glaucoma is very unusual.

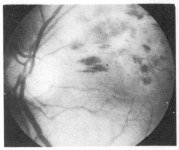

Branch retinal vein occlusion.

Occlusion of the central retinal artery

Clinical features

There is profound loss of vision and frequently light perception is absent. The pupil reacts poorly to light if at all. The retina is opalescent due to oedema and the retinal arterioles are threadlike and irregular. Transmission of the choroidal circulation at the fovea, where the retina is thin, gives the appearance of a cherry red spot. Optic atrophy develops after a few weeks.

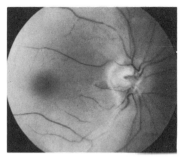

Central retinal artery occlusion.

Causes

1. Thrombosis in a central retinal artery damaged by arteriosclerosis or hypertension.
2. Emboli from atheromatous carotid arteries or diseased heart valves.
3. Inflammatory changes in the central retinal artery due to giant-cell arteritis. This is uncommon.

SLE, PAN, Syphilis

Management

Giant-cell arteritis as a possible cause should be excluded by measuring the erythrocyte sedimentation rate (*see* Chapter 28). If the cause is likely to be the result of embolus or thromobosis rapid reduction of the intraocular pressure (by digital massage, intravenous acetazolamide or paracentesis of the anterior chamber) within the first 2 hours may allow circulation to be re-established. Most patients arrive too late for such measures.

Cardiovascular assessment is required to determine the source of an embolus or cause of thrombosis. Anticoagulants and fibrinolytic agents are not useful. ✳

5% of pts c̄ Giant-Cell Arteritis → CRAO (c̄ Cherry Red Spot)

Vitreous haemorrhage

Clinical features

Haemorrhage into the vitreous may cause floaters or loss of vision. Examination with the ophthalmoscope reveals a partial or total loss of the red reflex from the fundus.

Smoke drifting across the sky

Causes

Bleeding from a retinal blood vessel into the vitreous gel. This occurs in:

1. Proliferative diabetic retinopathy.
2. Any other cause of retinal or optic disc *neovascularization*, e.g. branch retinal vein occlusion.
3. Spontaneous tearing of the retina which may precede retinal detachment.
4. Systemic hypertension.

Management

The cause must be identified and treated accordingly. If the haemorrhage is dense ultrasound examination may be necessary to ascertain if the retina is detached. If the haemorrhage fails to clear spontaneously within 6 months surgical removal of the vitreous (vitrectomy) may be necessary.

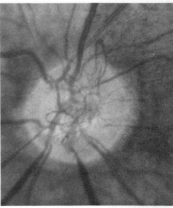

Optic disc neovascularization.

Retinal detachment

Retinal detachment is the separation of the two embryonic layers of the retina (the neuro-retina from the pigment epithelium) and not a separation of the retina from the choroid.

Causes

Primary retinal detachment is caused by a tear in the neuro-retina which allows fluid, derived from the vitreous, to lift it away from the underlying pigment epithelium. This condition is more common in myopic individuals and following cataract extraction. There is a 25% chance of the second eye being similarly affected.

Secondary retinal detachment may result from traction on the neuro-retina; this occurs most commonly in proliferative diabetic retinopathy. Separation of the two layers of the retina can also be caused by the accumulation of serous fluid which frequently accompanies malignant tumours of the choroid.

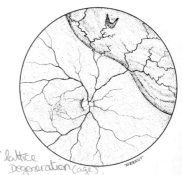

Retinal detachment.

Clinical features

A shadow appears in the field of vision and increases in size. A primary retinal detachment may be preceded by vitreous floaters and flashing lights before the shadow appears. This is caused by tearing of the retina.
The detached retina is elevated and grey in colour and may undulate with movement of the eye. The overlying retinal vessels appear dark and tortuous.

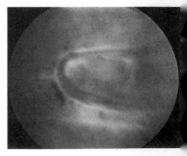

Retinal tear.

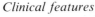

Careful examination of the retinal periphery may reveal a tear in the retina which is often horseshoe shaped.

Management

A primary retinal detachment is treated by identification and sealing of the retinal tear (*see* Chapter 35). A traction retinal detachment in diabetes requires treatment if the macula is affected or threatened. Elaborate vitreo-retinal surgery is necessary to remove the fibrous tissue and reattach the retina. Surgery is seldom indicated in secondary retinal detachment caused by a serous effusion.

Optic and retrobulbar neuritis

These conditions are essentially the same. The optic disc is swollen in optic neuritis but in retrobulbar neuritis the disc appears normal as the site of inflammation is more posterior.

Clinical features

Loss of central vision varies from mild to profound and characteristically there is a dull ache with pain on movement of the eye, especially elevation. The loss of vision may be temporarily aggravated by physical exertion or eating.

Typical findings include an afferent pupillary defect, a central scotoma and defective colour vision. In the acute phase the optic disc may appear swollen or normal but following recovery temporal pallor is common. Visually evoked responses recorded over the occipital cortex show an increased latency that persists after clinical recovery (*see* Chapter 33). This is almost pathognomonic of optic neuritis and retrobulbar neuritis.

The second eye may become involved, though seldom simultaneously, and repeated attacks are not uncommon.

Causes

Demyelination is by far the most common cause of optic and retrobulbar neuritis. Other signs and symptoms of multiple sclerosis may later develop.

Other causes of optic neuritis, such as syphilis and herpes zoster, are relatively uncommon.

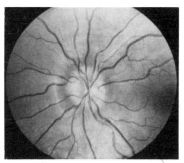
Swollen disc in optic neuritis.

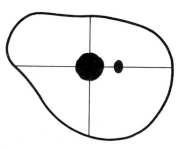
Central scotoma in optic neuritis.

Management

This is expectant. The majority of patients under the age of 45 will recover within 2 months and regain normal visual acuity. Recovery is less certain and may be incomplete in older patients.

Systemic steroids are of doubtful value. The recovery period may be shortened but the final visual outcome is unaffected.

If recovery is poor, and especially if the second eye is involved, optic nerve and chiasmal compression *must* be excluded as a cause for the visual loss.

Ischaemic optic neuropathy

→ Loss of upper ½ or Lower ½
= Altitudinal Vis field Defect

Clinical features

This affects the older age group; visual loss is often severe. An afferent pupillary defect is present and ophthalmoscopy reveals a pale swollen optic disc with small 'splinter' haemorrhages.

Causes

Occlusion of the *short posterior ciliary arteries* by:

1. Giant-cell (temporal) arteritis.
2. Arteriosclerotic or hypertensive vessel disease.

acute blood loss or Chr. ↓e Def Anaemia.

Management

Ischaemic optic neuropathy.

If giant-cell arteritis is diagnosed, systemic steroids, in high doses initially, must be given as a matter of urgency to prevent involvement of the second eye (*see* Chapter 28).

No treatment is effective in the non-arteritic form of the disease. Steroids, anticoagulants and vasodilators are not useful.

Choroiditis

Inflammation of the choroid may affect the vision through involvement of the overlying retina or adjacent optic nerve or by clouding of the vitreous.

Clinical features

Loss of vision in this condition usually occurs over a matter of hours or days. A focus of active choroiditis appears white and fluffy and the overlying vitreous is cloudy. Later, when the lesion is quiescent, there are varying degrees of scarring and pigmentation and the sclera may be exposed, appearing as a white patch.

Causes

1. Congenital toxoplasmosis (*see* Chapter 29).
2. Less commonly, tuberculosis, syphilis and, in the USA, histoplasmosis.
3. In many cases the cause is unknown.

Management

Treatment with systemic steroids may be necessary to suppress the inflammation and avoid retinal (especially macular) damage. Specific treatment may be indicated when the cause is known. Choroiditis is frequently a recurrent condition.

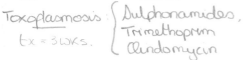

Toxoplasmosis : {Sulphonamides, Trimethoprim, Clindomycin
tx = 3 wks.

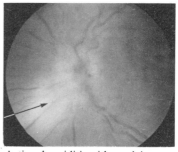

Active choroiditis with overlying vitreous haze.

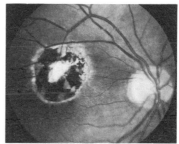

Chorioretinal scar of inactive toxoplasmosis.

Homonymous hemianopia

Not infrequently homonymous hemianopia (*see* Chapter 27) of sudden onset is interpreted by the patient as loss of vision in one eye. However, the visual acuity and pupil reactions are usually normal in both eyes. The nature of the visual loss is readily diagnosed by confrontation testing of the visual fields.

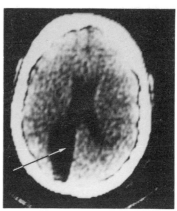

CT scan of left occipital infarct causing right homonymous hemianopia

Gradual loss of vision

Gradual loss of vision by its very nature is not dramatic. The underlying disease is usually *bilateral* though frequently asymmetric. Poor vision in one eye may only be noticed by the patient when the better eye is covered, the loss then appearing to be sudden in onset.

Gradual loss of vision may present as:

1. Reduction in visual acuity. The patient may complain of reading difficulty or the inability to recognize faces.
2. Diminished field of vision. Difficulty may be encountered with ball games or, if field loss is advanced, the patient may experience navigational difficulties.

Or, less often as:

3. Poor colour discrimination.
4. Impaired dark adaptation—night blindness.

A carefully taken history will often suggest the likely cause of the visual loss.

Causes of gradual loss of vision

The causes of gradual loss of vision include :

1. **Refractive errors**
2. **Cataract**
3. **Macular degeneration**
4. **Chronic glaucoma**
5. **Diabetic retinopathy**
6. **Retinitis pigmentosa**
7. **Malignant melanoma of the choroid**
8. **Optic nerve and chiasmal disease**

Refractive errors

Certain refractive errors present as gradual loss of vision and must be excluded before a pathological cause is sought. Myopia commonly develops in the early teens and difficulty reading the blackboard may be the first complaint. In older individuals hypermetropia that cannot be corrected by accommodation may present as deteriorating near vision. This also occurs in normal individuals in their mid forties (presbyopia).

Occasionally refractive errors are associated with or caused by *ocular disease*.

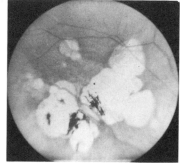

Degenerative myopia—chorioretinal atrophy.

Myopia

Degenerative myopia

Very high degrees of myopia (greater than 15 dioptres) are accompanied by degenerative retinal changes. These eyes are also more prone to develop glaucoma and cataract. Degenerative myopia is a significant cause of blind registration.

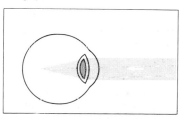

Nuclear sclerosis causing myopia.

Lenticular myopia

In old age sclerosis of the central part (nucleus) of the lens increases the refractive power of the eye (*see* Cataract, *below*).

Astigmatism

Progressive irregular astigmatism occurs in *keratoconus* (conical cornea). Contact lenses may provide adequate vision initially but corneal grafting is often required.

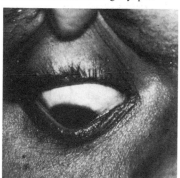

Keratoconus.

Cataract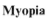

Cataract is one of the commonest causes of visual loss and is responsible for a high percentage of the patients referred for ophthalmic assessment.

The normal crystalline lens of the eye is optically clear. A lens that has become opaque is termed a cataract. Small opacities, commonly congenital, are frequently found in otherwise healthy eyes and do not merit the term cataract unless progressive or causing visual difficulty.

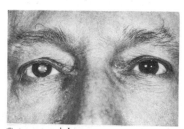

Cataract—right eye.

Symptoms

Gradual failure of Vision.
Uniocular Diplopia (ghosting)
Haloes (when look at Light)
Δ in colour values
(adventitious Myopia)

Signs
mild: Black Shaddow against
Red Reflex
adv: white opacity in pupil.

Causes and clinical features

1. Senile. The majority of cataracts occur in the elderly and are the result of biochemical changes within the lens which are poorly understood. Senile cataracts may take different forms and the position and density of the opacity determine the effect on vision. The common types of senile cataract are:

a. Cortical lens opacities. These are seen as black spokes against the red reflex with the ophthalmoscope. Vision is distorted and the patient is troubled by glare.

b. Nuclear sclerosis. The centre of the lens becomes progressively yellow then brown. Myopia is caused in the early stages resulting in deterioration of distance vision while sometimes allowing the patient to discard reading glasses.

c. Posterior subcapsular opacification. This is seen as a central black spot against the red reflex. Vision may be little affected until the pupil constricts, as in reading or bright sunlight.

d. Mature cataract. There is total opacification of the lens which results in a white pupil. Vision is reduced to perception of hand movements or a light.

2. Congenital. Congenital cataract may be hereditary, the result of intra-uterine infection or due to a metabolic disorder.

if Bilat
⇒ Early
Surgery.
Unilat - not urgent, nor v. successful.

3. Metabolic. These are uncommon. True diabetic cataract occurs in young insulin-dependent diabetics and may present as sudden deterioration of vision. Galactosaemia causes an 'oil drop' lens opacity in infants which is reversible in the early stages if the condition is diagnosed and treated.

Hypoparathyroidism is a rare cause of cataract.

4. Drug induced. Systemic steroids given in a dose greater than 10 mg of prednisolone daily for more than a year may cause a characteristic posterior subcapsular cataract.

5. Trauma. Both sudden and gradual opacification of the lens may follow blunt or penetrating trauma to the eye.

6. Chronic uveitis. Longstanding intraocular inflammation usually results in secondary cataract formation. This is particularly common in juvenile rheumatoid arthritis (Still's disease).

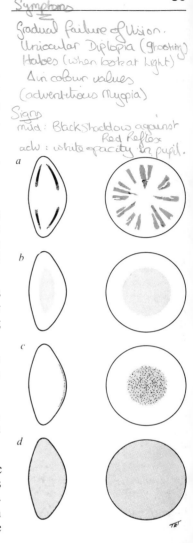

a

b

c

d

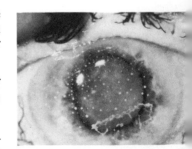

Cataract secondary to chronic iritis. The white spots are keratic precipitates.

Management

Treatment is surgical by removal of the cataract and correction of the optical defect caused by absence of the lens (aphakia) (*see* Chapter 35).

[handwritten: Yag laser.]

*[handwritten top right: Indications for surgery
1. Unable to work
2. " " Read.
3. Loss of Vision.]*

Macular degeneration

Macular degeneration is the commonest cause of blindness in the developed world among patients over the age of 65.

[handwritten: 27% of Causes of Blindness in UK]

Clinical features

In the early stages of macular degeneration objects are distorted and straight lines appear bent. Reading is affected early on. Eventually a central scotoma develops with reduction of visual acuity to less than 6/60. Peripheral vision is unaffected allowing continuing mobility.

Ophthalmoscopically there is disturbance of the normal macular architecture. Usually this can only be seen through the dilated pupil.

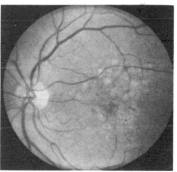

'Dry' senile macular degeneration.

Causes

1. Senile macular degeneration. The great majority of patients presenting with macular degeneration are elderly. There are two distinct ophthalmoscopic appearances.

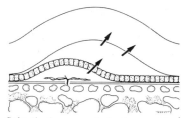

Subretinal neovascularization. *[handwritten: = Wet .]*

a. 'Dry'. The pigment epithelium of the retina is disturbed, giving rise to dark clumps and intervening areas of choroidal exposure. Refractile bodies are frequently present.

[handwritten: ⇒: early laser tx]

b. 'Wet'. Subretinal neovascularization from the choroid results in haemorrhage and exudate leading to scar formation (disciform macular degeneration). Colloid bodies are almost invariably present (*see* Chapter 16). *[handwritten: Hyaline Bodies due to degeneration in "Bruch's" Memb. ≡ "Drusen" Argoid streaks]*

2. Hereditary. This usually presents in the second and third decades. Electrodiagnostic assessment of retinal function may allow early diagnosis before the appearance of typical ophthalmoscopic features.

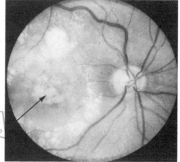

Disciform degeneration (arrowed) surrounded by exudate.

3. Drug induced. Chloroquine and derivatives may cause a pigmentary maculopathy of 'bull's eye' appearance. This is related to the total dose of the drug given. Irreversible damage to central vision may occur unless the earliest changes are detected by regular examination of the central visual field and the drug is stopped.

4. High Myopes — → Defects in Bruchs Memb .

Management

Argon L

There is no treatment for the 'dry' type of senile macular degeneration. In the 'wet' type early diagnosis of a subretinal neovascular membrane by fluorescein angiography may allow laser treatment and prevent the development of a disciform macular degeneration. For patients with established macular degeneration low vision aids are helpful in addition to the provision of large print books and 'Talking Books.'

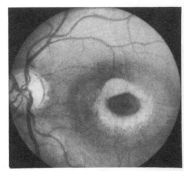

Chloroquine 'bull's eye' maculopathy.

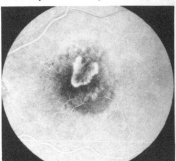

Fluorescein angiogram of macula showing neovascular membrane.

Chronic glaucoma

(i) ↑ IOP
(ii) Disc Cupping
(iii) Visual field loss.

The term 'glaucoma' implies raised intraocular pressure. There are many different types of which the commonest is *chronic open angle glaucoma*. This is uncommon under the age of 40 but is a major blinding disease in the elderly.

Clinical features

Chronic glaucoma is an asymptomatic disease. Loss of vision is *painless and gradual*. Central vision is preserved until late in the course of the disease. Diagnosis is made on the basis of three characteristic findings:

1. The intraocular pressure is raised above the normal range of 10–21 mmHg. It can be accurately measured by applanation tonometry. This involves the use of an instrument which flattens a small, predetermined area of the anaesthetized cornea. The force applied is proportional to the intraocular pressure and is read directly from a calibrated scale.

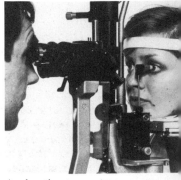

Applanation tonometry.

2. Pathological cupping of the optic disc. There is gradual loss of nerve fibres at the optic disc together with glial supporting cells and capillaries. This results in a pale disc with an enlarged cup. There is preferential loss of nerve fibres at the upper and lower poles of the disc.

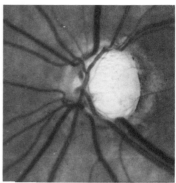

3. Visual field loss. There is a characteristic pattern of field loss in chronic glaucoma:

a. The first defect is usually a paracentral scotoma lying above or below fixation at a distance of 10–20°.

b. The defect slowly enlarges to form an arcuate scotoma which runs into the blind spot. At the same time there is contraction of the peripheral field, particularly on the nasal side.

Glaucomatous cupping of the optic disc.

c. In time upper and lower arcuate scotomata meet to leave a central island of vision often only a few degrees across. A temporal area of field may remain after this central island is lost.

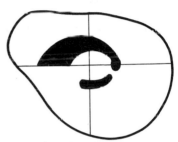

Arcuate scotomata.

Causes

In chronic open angle glaucoma the drainage angle of the eye is normal in appearance. The outflow of aqueous from the anterior chamber of the eye is impaired by an alteration in the function of the trabecular meshwork which overlies the canal of Schlemm. The cause is unknown but there is a familial tendency.

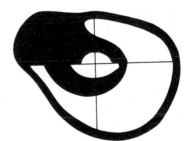

Nasal field loss.

Management

Progressive visual field loss can be prevented by lowering the intraocular pressure to within the normal range. This can be achieved by:

1. Medical treatment using one or more of the following drugs:

a. Pilocarpine drops 1–4% which act through the ciliary muscle to open the drainage channels. Pupillary constriction is an unwanted side effect of treatment.

b. Timolol drops 0·25–0·5% reduce the rate of formation of aqueous humour.

c. Adrenaline drops 0·5–2% increase the outflow of aqueous humour from the eye but the mechanism of action is uncertain. The pressure-lowering effect is enhanced by the simultaneous use of *guanethidine* drops.

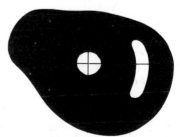

Tunnel vision and temporal island.

Progressive visual field loss, in glaucoma—right eye.

d. Acetazolamide tablets 250 mg reduce the rate of aqueous formation.

2. *Laser treatment*. If the drainage angle is open the application of minute laser burns to the trabecular meshwork results in increased aqueous outflow. This procedure is known as *laser trabeculoplasty*. (argon laser)

3. *Surgical drainage*. A portion of sclera adjacent the cornea is removed to create a fistula. The commonest operation of this type is a *trabeculectomy* (*see* Chapter 35).

The patient with chronic glaucoma must remain under observation for life. Treatment is regularly monitored by applanation tonometry and perimetry. Success is gauged by the degree to which further visual field loss can be prevented.

Diabetic retinopathy

Diabetic retinopathy is a major cause of visual loss. Mild or 'background' disease is compatible with normal vision but exudative changes at the macula or the development of proliferative retinopathy result in progressive loss of vision (*see* Chapter 25).

Retinitis pigmentosa

A Dom / A. Recess / X-linked.

This disease is uncommon but of importance because of its early onset and relentless progression towards blindness. In fact it is a genetically determined *group* of diseases in some of which a disorder of lipid metabolism has been incriminated. There is no inflammatory element in the disease process and the term 'retinitis' is a misnomer.

? abn of Rodopsin formation.

Clinical features
Typically the patient complains of poor vision at night (night blindness). Ophthalmoscopy reveals pigmentary degeneration of the retina in which clumps of pigment assume a 'bone corpuscle' pattern. The retinal blood vessels are attenuated and there is a waxy pallor of the optic disc. There is progressive loss of the peripheral visual field leading to 'tunnel vision' and eventual blindness.

constricted-narrows

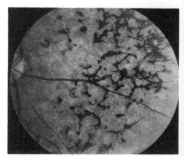

Retinitis pigmentosa.

O.D. Hyaline material on surface or Buried just beneath surface.
—called DRUSEN. (≠ Macular Oedema).

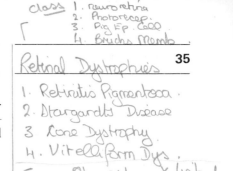

Handwritten margin notes:

class 1. neuro retina
2. Photorecep.
3. Pig Ep. Cell
4. Bruchs Memb.

Retinal Dystrophies
1. Retinitis Pigmentosa.
2. Stargardts Disease
3. Cone Dystrophy
4. Vitelliform Dys.
5. ~ Choroid – X-linked
  ε Choroideraemia peripheral Vis
6. Gyrate Atrophy – Can be .
– def of ornithine. (:. gwe to child.
Periph Areas – later Central. (v. early on).

Retinitis pigmentosa may be part of a more wide-spread disorder or syndrome e.g. Laurence–Moon–Biedl syndrome, which consists of obesity, gonadal hypoplasia and retinitis pigmentosa.

Management

There is *no treatment of proven benefit* in halting the progression of this disease. Genetic counselling is of great importance.

Malignant melanoma of the choroid

Clinical features

Almost invariably unilateral. A malignant melanoma of the choroid may present as either loss of visual field or loss of acuity depending on the site of the tumour. Ophthalmoscopy reveals a 'solid' retinal detachment which is usually pigmented.

Differential diagnosis

Pigmented choroidal lesions are common, but the vast majority are benign naevi; the hallmarks of malignancy are elevation and progressive enlargement.

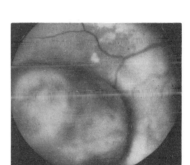

Malignant melanoma of the choroid.

Other lesions which may be confused with malignant melanoma of the choroid are disciform degeneration of the macula, choroidal haemangioma and secondary choroidal tumours, particularly from carcinoma of the breast.

Treatment

The beneficial effects of removal of an eye with a malignant melanoma are uncertain and if the tumour is small and useful vision remains a conservative approach is often adopted. The liver is the commonest site of metastases; these may appear many years after the discovery of the primary tumour. If the tumour is increasing in size removal of the eye (enucleation) may be undertaken. Local excision of small malignant melanomas is feasible.

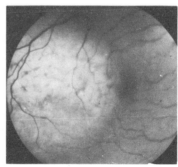

Choroidal secondary from breast carcinoma.

Optic nerve and chiasmal disease

It is important to remember the possibility of orbital and intracranial disease as a cause of gradual loss of

vision. Careful examination of the visual fields is essential when no ocular disease can be found to account for loss of vision. Disease of the optic nerve or chiasm usually results in:
1. Decreased visual acuity
2. Visual field loss   — Bitemporal Hemianopia '
3. Optic atrophy

Causes (see also Chapter 27)

1. *Chiasmal compression*, particularly from pituitary tumours and meningiomas.

2. *Nutritional amblyopia*. This condition is usually related to heavy drinking and/or smoking and is often referred to as *tobacco-alcohol amblyopia*. A diet poor in vitamin B complex is a contributary factor.

There is bilateral loss of central vision and visual acuity may be less than 6/60. Examination of the visual fields reveals central scotomata which encompass the blind spot and fixation (centro-caecal). Colour discrimination is reduced and there may be pallor of the optic discs. A similar condition occurs in pernicious anaemia (*see* Chapter 30).

Treatment consists of vitamin B supplements, in particular injections of hydroxocobalamin, and, ideally, withdrawal of alcohol and tobacco.

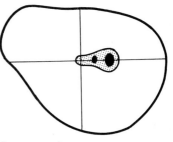

Centro-caecal scotoma.

3. *Tumours of the optic nerve* such as meningioma or glioma are a rare cause of gradual loss of vision in one eye.

Transient loss of vision

4

Sudden loss or blurring of vision with return of normal function within a few minutes or hours is not uncommon. A careful history and examination will usually indicate the likely cause and need for special investigations.

Migraine

The visual symptoms which precede classical migraine headache consist of brightly coloured flashes (teichopsia) with a typically zig-zag or castellated pattern (fortification spectrum). The visual symptoms last for up to 30 min and are often accompanied by loss of vision which may affect the central or peripheral fields and be unilateral or bilateral. Homonymous field loss is common.

The repeated and paroxysmal nature of the attacks combined with a positive family history confirm the diagnosis and further investigations are usually unnecessary.

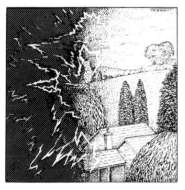

Visual aura and field loss in migraine.

Subacute glaucoma

An attack of acute angle closure glaucoma (*see* Chapter 7) may be preceded by one or several episodes of subacute glaucoma. Women are affected more commonly than men and the episodes occur especially at night. The vision becomes blurred in one eye which aches. The *rapid* rise in intraocular pressure causes corneal oedema which produces coloured rainbow haloes around lights. The attacks usually resolve with sleep.

It is important to recognize the problem at this stage since an acute attack can be prevented by peripheral iridectomy. Some patients are incorrectly diagnosed as suffering from migraine until, eventually, a full blown attack of acute glaucoma develops.

Retinal emboli and temporary vascular occlusion

Patients may present with a history of sudden loss of vision in one eye which is altitudinal and described as 'like a shutter coming down'. This may last for a few seconds to 2 or 3 minutes with complete recovery. The term 'amaurosis fugax' is used to describe this fleeting blindness.

Amaurosis fugax is caused by :

1. *Emboli* from the heart and great vessels of the neck.
2. *Carotid artery stenosis*.
3. *Vertebrobasilar ischaemia*.

The commonest underlying pathology is atheroma which is discussed in Chapter 26.

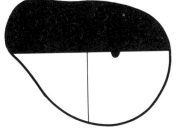

Altitudinal visual field loss.

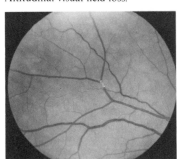

Retinal embolus.

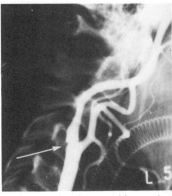

Angiogram showing carotid stenosis.

Papilloedema

Patients with moderate papilloedema due to raised intracranial pressure experience no visual symptoms as a result of the disc swelling but when the papilloedema is severe they may complain of fleeting loss of vision, often in both eyes, lasting for only a few seconds. This indicates that the circulation within the optic nerve is severely embarrassed and the pressure should be relieved as a matter of urgency to prevent the development of optic atrophy and blindness.

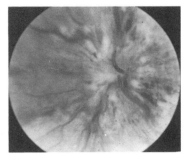

Severe papilloedema.

Functional loss of vision

5

Loss of vision in the absence of organic disease is termed 'functional'. Diagnosis and management may present considerable problems.

Hysteria

Hysterical loss of vision may present as total blindness, decreased vision in one or both eyes or visual field loss. There may appear to have been a sudden precipitating cause, such as a blow to the head, but frequently the loss appears to be spontaneous in onset.

Clinical features

The patient is usually calm though concerned. Occasionally there is total indifference. Examination reveals no physical abnormality of the eyes and in particular the pupil reactions are normal.

If total blindness is claimed a difference may be noted in the patient's behaviour, for example in navigating a room full of furniture, depending on whether the patient is aware of the presence of an observer.

Decreased visual acuity in one or both eyes tends to be inconsistent and only the top letter on the Snellen chart may be read, irrespective of the distance. Visual field loss is similarly inconsistent even during the course of a single examination.

Differential diagnosis

1. RETROBULBAR NEURITIS

The eye with visual loss from retrobulbar neuritis may appear normal but careful examination of the pupil reflexes will usually reveal an afferent pupillary defect.

The central scotoma is consistent in size. Confirmation of the diagnosis can be made by investigation of the visually evoked responses (*see* Chapter 2).

2. AMBLYOPIA

The vision in one eye may fail to develop normally during early childhood in the presence of a significant unilateral refractive error or squint (*see* Chapter 19). The resultant poor vision may not be noticed until later childhood or even adult life when it may appear to be sudden in onset. The absence of any demonstrable physical abnormality together with the finding of a unilateral refractive error (usually hypermetropia) or a small squint confirms the diagnosis.

3. CORTICAL BLINDNESS

Cortical blindness, usually resulting from bilateral infarction of the occipital lobes, can be particularly difficult to diagnose. Pupil reactions are normal and the patient may be indifferent to the visual loss or even deny it. Confirmation of the diagnosis is obtained by the absence of visually evoked responses or the demonstration of occipital infarction on CT scanning.

4. MALINGERING

Poor vision, either in the absence of physical findings or out of proportion to ocular disease, may be claimed for the purposes of personal gain. If unilateral it is easy to demonstrate normal, or better-than-claimed vision, by using methods to assess vision which do not allow the patient to appreciate which eye is being tested.

Management

Hysterical blindness is usually impossible to treat though the underlying cause may be identified by psychiatric assessment. Patients who are hysterically blind are severely incapacitated and may be registered as blind. Spontaneous conversion of these individuals back to normal sight is responsible for the vast majority of 'miracle cures' of blindness reported in the popular press.

Functional loss of vision occurs not uncommonly in schoolchildren, particularly girls. The visual loss is usually confined to one eye and is seldom incapacitating. It is difficult to know whether the visual loss represents a mild form of hysteria or malingering but a problem at home or at school can often be identified. Spontaneous improvement is the rule and all that is required is explanation to the parents and reassurance to the child. Psychiatric investigation rarely seems to be indicated.

Convergence spasm

This condition is usually a form of hysterical reaction. The spasm involves convergence, accommodation and miosis of the pupil. The patient complains of diplopia, blurred vision and discomfort. The reaction is brought on by looking at an object, shining a light in the eyes or even by touching the lids.

Treatment for this distressing condition is difficult. Atropine drops may help by paralysing the ciliary muscle. Occasionally, psychiatric assessment is required but patients often exchange this problem for another.

Blindness 6

In order to be registered as blind in the United Kingdom a person must be 'so blind as to be unable to perform any work for which eyesight is essential'. In practice a person with visual acuity below 3/60 is regarded as blind but a person with normal acuity and severe contraction of the visual fields may also be eligible for registration.

Individuals with poor sight who do not qualify as blind may be registered as 'partially sighted'. This is of particular importance to children who may require special schooling and adults in need of retraining for another job.

It should be noted that loss of vision in one eye does not mean that the individual is 'partially sighted'.

Blindness in the developed world

The commonest cause of blindness in persons over the age of 65 is *macular degeneration*. In the younger age group *diabetic retinopathy* is now the leading cause. Other serious causes of blindness include *glaucoma*, *myopic* and other *retinal degenerations*, *trauma* and *congenital abnormalities*.

Cataract is a frequent cause of loss of vision but with few exceptions is treatable. Patients with cataract who are registered blind usually have coexisting, untreatable ocular disease.

[handwritten margin notes: ≥65 ~ Macular Degeneration; younger - Diabetic Retinopathy; also]

Blindness in underdeveloped countries

There are some 40 million blind people in underdeveloped countries throughout the world.

Many are blind from diseases which are endemic in certain areas.

The major causes of blindness in the under-developed world are:

Trachoma
Xerophthalmia
Onchocerciasis
Cataract
Chronic glaucoma

Leprosy and measles are other important causes (*see* Chapter 29).

Trachoma

Trachoma is the most important single cause of preventable blindness. One hundred million people are affected by the disease of whom at least 2 million are blind. It is prevalent throughout much of the developing world and is due in large part to poverty, overcrowding and poor hygiene. It is by far the most common cause of blindness in North Africa and the Middle East.

The disease is caused by infection with *Chlamydia trachomatis*. It is spread by flies which feed on infected excreta and which also transmit the organism directly from eye to eye. A chronic follicular conjunctivitis leads to conjunctival and corneal scarring and distortion of the eyelids with entropion and trichiasis.

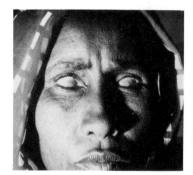
Trachomatous corneal scarring.

Treatment

Active trachoma can be effectively treated with tetracycline ointment. When lid scarring is established surgery is required to correct entropion and trichiasis; corneal grafting may improve vision.

Prevention

The main hope of reducing the incidence of blindness from trachoma lies in prevention. This may be achieved by the widespread use of topical antibiotics as a prophylactic measure and improved hygiene.

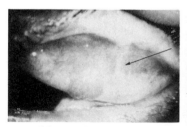
Upper lid everted to show conjunctival scarring.

Xerophthalmia

Xerophthalmia is a major cause of childhood blindness in Asia and to a lesser extent Africa and Latin America. It is particularly prevalent in Indonesia. Each year a quarter of a million children are affected by this disease.

Xerophthalmia is caused by vitamin A deficiency but virtually all children who are blinded are severely malnourished. The earliest clinical manifestation is *night blindness*. Conjunctival xerosis (dryness) is indicated by the presence of *Bitôt's spots* next to the cornea. These have a 'foamy' appearance. *Corneal xerosis* is seen initially as mild haziness inferiorly. Corneal ulceration may supervene with full thickness corneal dissolution known as *keratomalacia.*

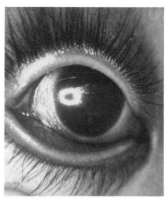

Conjunctival and corneal xerosis.

Treatment

Vitamin A therapy and a protein-rich diet are essential. Secondary bacterial infection in corneal xerosis requires topical antibiotics. The clinical response to treatment is rapid but keratomalacia results in permanent corneal scarring.

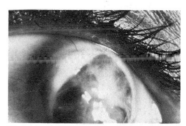

Keratomalacia.

Prevention

Nutritional blindness can be prevented by ensuring that every child has an adequate intake of vitamin A. This can be achieved in a number of ways including the distribution of supplemental vitamin A to children in high risk areas, the fortification of processed foods and the consumption of local foods rich in vitamin A or its precursor, beta-carotene.

Onchocerciasis

It is estimated that 20–30 million people, mainly in tropical West Africa and Central and South America are infected by this parasitic disease which is also known as '*river blindness*'. A million persons are blind from this condition.

The black fly, which is found alongside running waters, is host to the *Onchocerca volvulus* worm which migrates as microfilariae throughout the human body. These invade every structure of the eye causing corneal scarring, chronic iritis and chorioretinal degeneration.

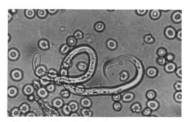

Onchocerca volvulus.

Cataract and optic atrophy may develop. Damage is caused both by living microfilariae and through immunological reaction to the dead organisms.

Treatment

There is no effective treatment of the established disease. Prevention, by eradication of the vector, is difficult; spraying of the rivers with insecticide has to be continued for many years.

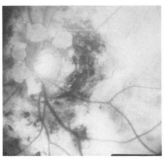

Chorioretinal degeneration in onchocerciasis.

Cataract and glaucoma in the under-developed world

Millions are blind from cataract, particularly in the rural areas of the Indian Subcontinent (5 million) and Africa (3 million). This is due solely to the lack of medical facilities.

The establishment of mobile eye camps is the only practical solution to this problem at the present time. One eye surgeon may carry out as many as 100 cataract operations in a day, all under local anaesthesia, and the success rate is high. Literally hundreds of thousands of people have had their sight restored in this way.

Chronic glaucoma is prevalent in all communities and affects the elderly especially. Early detection of the disease and its control pose great difficulties in widely scattered communities with poor medical facilities.

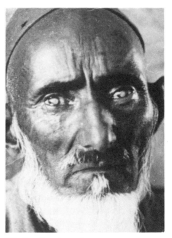

Bilateral cataract.

Section 2
Ocular pain and discomfort

The acute red eye   7

The acute red eye is due to inflammation of the anterior part of the eye which causes a variable degree of pain and, depending on the tissue involved, discharge, photophobia, loss of vision and pupillary abnormality.

Δ° of - Pain
Discharge
Photophobia.
Vision . Loss .
pupillary alt (N)

By contrast, inflammation of the choroid and retina causes painless loss of vision in an eye that appears externally normal.

Ocular injury frequently results in a red eye but is dealt with separately under Trauma. Acute inflammations of the eyelids and other structures surrounding the eye are considered in Section 3.

Causes of the acute red eye

Common causes of the acute red eye include:

Conjunctivitis
Keratitis—inflammation of the cornea
Iritis
Acute glaucoma
Episcleritis   *— (space between Conjunctiva + Sclera).*
Scleritis

One of the commonest causes of a *suddenly* red eye is *subconjunctival haemorrhage*. There is usually no difficulty in distinguishing this from the more important inflammatory causes but the appearance may alarm the patient and is included here for the purpose of differential diagnosis.

Conjunctivitis

Conjunctivitis is usually a bilateral disease. There are many causes but the great majority are the result of acute infection or allergy. Specific symptoms, signs and management depend on the exact cause.

Bacterial

Clinical features

There is mucopurulent discharge and the lashes are stuck together on waking. The patient experiences a gritty discomfort rather than pain and any blurring of vision is due to mucopus in the tear film which clears with blinking.

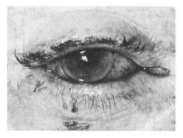

Causes

A wide variety of bacteria may be responsible. Common organisms include *Staphylococcus aureus*, *Streptococcus pyogenes*, haemophilus and coliforms.

Bacterial conjunctivitis.

Management

Broad-spectrum antibiotic drops, e.g. chloramphenicol, must be instilled frequently in the acute stage of the disease. Culture of the responsible organism seldom plays an important part in the management of acute conjunctivitis.

Chlamydial

These obligate intracellular bacteria cause trachoma, a chronic blinding conjunctivitis, in many areas of the underdeveloped world (*see* Chapter 6).

In the developed world chlamydial infection causes acute conjunctivitis in young adults and neonates.

The acute form of the disease, known as inclusion conjunctivitis, may present in one or both eyes with marked lid swelling, discomfort and hypertrophy of the lymph follicles. Conjunctival scarring and permanent corneal changes, however, are rare. Tetracycline applied topically as an ointment is effective in treatment; systemic tetracycline may need to be given if there is a genital reservoir of the disease (*see* Chapter 29).

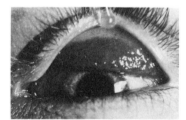

Inclusion conjunctivitis—follicular hypertrophy of upper tarsal conjunctiva.

Viral

Clinical features

There is often considerable discomfort accompanied by a profuse watery discharge. The cornea is frequently involved as well (keratoconjunctivitis) with slight blurring of vision. The punctate corneal lesions,

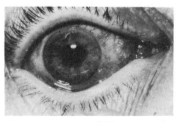

Adenovirus conjunctivitis.

however, are difficult to see without suitable magnification. The diagnosis is often made by the presence of tarsal conjunctival follicles and ⅍ preauricular lymphadenopathy.

Causes

Adenovirus infection is by far the most common cause of sporadic and epidemic viral conjunctivitis. There are many different serotypes and there may be associated upper respiratory tract infection.

Management

There is no specific treatment for adenovirus conjunctivitis. The condition is self-limiting with resolution in 2–3 weeks though corneal lesions may persist for months.

Allergic

Clinical features

The predominant symptom is intense irritation and itching of the eye. Oedema of the conjunctiva ~ noticeable. (chemosis) may be more noticeable than hyperaemia (mild) which is often mild in relation to the symptoms.

Causes

1. ATOPIC

Pollen hypersensitivity (hay fever) is the commonest cause of allergic conjunctivitis.

2. CONTACT

Usually the result of allergy to eye drops or the preservatives they contain. Characteristically there is associated dermatitis of the eyelids.

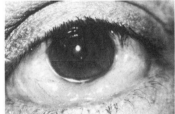
Chemosis in allergic conjunctivitis.

3. VERNAL

A recurrent seasonal conjunctivitis with distinctive marked papillary proliferation of the upper tarsal conjunctiva. The eyes are chronically inflamed with stringy mucoid discharge. There is a frequent association with eczema and asthma.

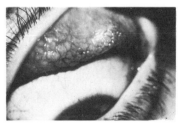
Papillary hypertrophy in vernal conjunctivitis.

Management
1. ATOPIC

Antihistamine drops and tablets. Identification of the antigen followed by desensitization is occasionally helpful.

2. CONTACT

Identification and removal of the irritant.

3. VERNAL

Topical steroids and sodium cromoglycate drops.

Keratitis

The cornea is an avascular, transparent structure. Inflammation results in loss of clarity caused initially by cellular infiltration and oedema and later by scarring. Reflex hyperaemia is most marked in the circumcorneal region. The rich sensory nerve supply of the cornea makes keratitis a painful condition.

Keratitis may be caused by a variety of bacterial, viral or fungal organisms or may be non-infective. Infective keratitis is usually, though not invariably, unilateral.

Causes
infections,
Tear film Disorder
Dystrophies,
Injuries, (hypopia
*   — c-lens).*
Exposure. — ↑ UV light
Neurotrophic.

Bacterial

Clinical features

The eye is red and painful with mucopurulent discharge. The resultant corneal ulcer is easily seen and appears white due to cellular infiltration of the corneal stroma. Pus cells accumulate in the anterior chamber and may form a white fluid level (*hypopyon*).

Causes

A break in the corneal epithelium is necessary for infection to become established. This is frequently traumatic but may be secondary to inadequate corneal protection or other corneal disease. Responsible organisms include *Staph. aureus, Strep. pneumococcus*, pseudomonas and enterobacteria. *Haemophilus. –(–ve)*
(-ve)   *(-ve)*

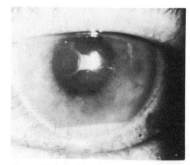

Bacterial keratitis with hypopyon formation.

Management

1. Identification of the infecting organism by Gram stain and culture.
2. Intensive topical antibiotics. *esp. Chloramphenicol / Gentamycin.*
3. Atropine drops to relieve associated ciliary and iris spasm.

Viral

Clinical features

There is typically a foreign body sensation and lacrimation.

Causes

1. HERPES SIMPLEX   *ulcers : Adults 20-50 yrs.*

This is by far the most common and serious cause of viral keratitis. Initially the disease is limited to the corneal epithelium with the formation of a dendritic ulcer. This may be difficult to see without the use of fluorescein and magnification. The majority of dendritic ulcers heal without serious sequelae but some progress to involve the corneal stroma with subsequent vascularization and scarring. Circumscribed ('disciform') keratitis and anterior uveitis occasionally occur as an immune reaction to the virus.

Herpes simplex keratitis is usually unilateral though frequently recurrent (*see* Chapter 29).

→ Metaherpetic Keratitis : (neurotrophisms).

2. HERPES ZOSTER

This can cause epithelial disease or neurotrophic keratitis which may result in severe corneal damage. Chickenpox rarely causes keratitis (*see* Chapter 29).

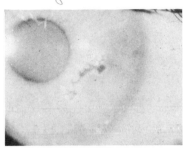

Dendritic corneal ulcer—stained with fluorescein.

H. simplex type I

1. Dendritic ulcer   90-95%
2. Disciform Keratitis   5%

1+2 may → Metaherpetic Keratitis.
⌐ Sterile Chr. Ker.

Management

Herpes simplex keratitis is treated by the use of topical antiviral agents such as idoxuridine, vidarabine and acyclovir. Topical steroids must *not* be used in the treatment of epithelial herpes simplex keratitis because, though they provide symptomatic relief, virus proliferation is enhanced and corneal perforation may occur. The use of topical steroids in the treatment of other types of viral keratitis may be necessary but requires specialist supervision.

Acyclovir : (ointment)
5 / Day   - 1wk.
± Dil of Pupil.

(may use steroids in Disciform)
(ē acyclovir)
~ may → Amoeboid ulcer
(Shape)
tx - As above

H. Zoster
Tx : Topical - Antibiotic ± Steroid
± Acyclovir
Systemic - ? Acyclovir?
Analgesia
(1) Anticonvulsants -
Na⁺ valproate
Carbamazepine
(2) Antidepressants
- TCA.
Does not respond to opioids.

Fungal

Fungal keratitis is relatively uncommon. The clinical picture is similar to that produced by bacteria but the progress of the disease is usually less dramatic and 'satellite' lesions may develop as the fungal hyphae spread through the corneal stroma. Hypopyon formation is common. Management consists of identification of the organism from scrapings and by culture and treatment with topical antifungal agents e.g. fluorocytosine. *Candida albicans* and aspergillus species are the commonest causes of fungal keratitis.

Tear film Disorder = Keratoconj. sicca
Dystrophy.
Injury
Exposure   Neurotrophic

Non-infective keratitis

Transient but very painful corneal damage may follow
exposure to high doses of ultraviolet light or the
overwearing of hard contact lenses. The latter is the
result of epithelial hypoxia. Treatment is symptomatic;
padding of the eyes and instillation of homatropine
drops help relieve discomfort but repeated use of
anaesthetic drops should be avoided (*see* Chapter 36).

Acute iritis

The uvea is the vascular coat of the eye comprising the
iris, ciliary body and choroid. Inflammation may
involve one or more parts of the uvea.

Anterior uveitis predominantly involves the iris, but
the ciliary body is frequently involved at the same time
(iridocyclitis).

Posterior uveitis or choroiditis causes blurring of
vision but no redness or pain.

Clinical features

Acute iritis is usually unilateral. However, the disease
is often recurrent and both eyes may be affected at
different times. There is pain, photophobia and a
slight to moderate reduction in visual acuity. The
pupil is smaller than the unaffected side and redness
of the eye is most marked in the circumcorneal region.

Diagnosis is dependent upon slit-lamp examination
of the eye. Cells and protein 'flare' are visible as the
slit beam of light illuminates the anterior chamber.
Aggregates of cells on the posterior corneal surface,
called keratic precipitates (KP), may be seen and, if the
iritis is severe, a hypopyon may form.

Causes

The iris may become a target site for circulating
immune complexes; iritis then reflects a disturbed
immune system and not a primary disease of the
eye. It is frequently associated with diseases such
as ankylosing spondylitis, Reiter's syndrome and
Behçet's syndrome in which abnormalities of the HLA
system are recognized.

Acute iritis also occurs in sarcoidosis (usually
bilateral) and secondary syphilis but *frequently no
cause or association can be found.*

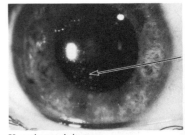

Keratic precipitates.

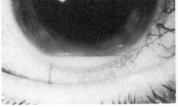

Hypopyon iritis.

Management

Topical steroids are used to suppress and shorten the course of the inflammation. Prednisolone, betamethasone and dexamethasone drops are used, sometimes as frequently as every hour depending on the severity of the disease.

Atropine drops are used to dilate the pupil so preventing the development of adhesions between the iris and lens (posterior synechiae). Atropine also relieves pain, due to spasm of the ciliary body, by paralysing the muscle (cycloplegia).

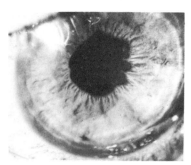

Posterior synechiae.

Chronic Iritis

In chronic iritis pain and redness are often minimal and may be absent. Posterior synechiae, however, are common and large keratic precipitates may be visible to the naked eye. Causes include juvenile rheumatoid arthritis (Still's disease), leprosy and tuberculosis.

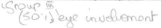
Group III
(50·1) eye involvement

Acute glaucoma

Clinical features

Acute glaucoma, a condition in which the intraocular pressure rapidly rises to high levels, occurs more commonly in women than in men. It is unusual under the age of 45. Symptoms include decreased vision, often to the level of counting fingers or worse, and severe pain described as a boring ache in and around the eye. Constitutional upset with nausea and vomiting is common.

The signs of acute glaucoma are diagnostic. In addition to the intense engorgement of the conjunctival and episcleral vessels there is corneal oedema with loss of the normal bright reflex from the corneal surface and the pupil is fixed, semi-dilated and often slightly oval in shape.

An acute attack of glaucoma may be preceded by one or more subacute attacks (*see* Chapter 4).

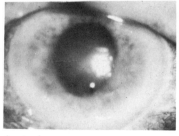

Acute glaucoma.

Causes

The predisposed eye has a shallow anterior chamber and narrow angle. This occurs most commonly in the elderly hypermetrope.

An acute attack is precipitated by partial dilatation of the pupil which causes :

1. Increased pressure in the posterior chamber of the

eye, between iris and lens, because aqueous flow through the pupil is restricted. This pushes the peripheral iris forwards against the trabecular meshwork of the drainage angle.

2. Crowding of the already narrow angle by iris.

The net result is angle closure and a dramatic rise in intraocular pressure from the normal level of about 15 mmHg to 60 + mmHg.

The initiating pupil dilatation may be caused by poor illumination, fear or apprehension, or drugs. The risk of *systemic* atropine-like drugs precipitating acute glaucoma is, however, low.

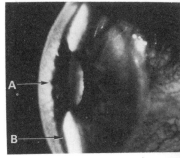

Acute glaucoma—optical section showing corneal oedema (A) and very shallow anterior chamber (B).

Management

1. *The initial treatment* of acute glaucoma is medical. The aim is to lower rapidly the intraocular pressure and constrict the pupil. Acetazolamide is given orally or intravenously to reduce the rate of formation of aqueous humour and pilocarpine drops are instilled to constrict the pupil. Anti-emetics and analgesics are given as necessary. Hyperosmotic agents, such as mannitol and glycerol which reduce the volume of the intraocular fluids, are given if the intraocular pressure does not fall within a few hours.

2. The *definitive treatment* is surgical. A *peripheral iridectomy* (or laser iridotomy) is carried out to allow free flow of aqueous from the posterior to the anterior chamber of the eye and widen the peripheral angle. Prophylactic iridectomy is recommended for the fellow eye.

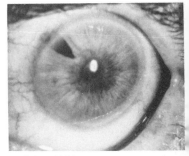

Peripheral iridectomy.

Episcleritis

The loose connective tissue between conjunctiva and sclera has a rich vascular supply. The episclera diminishes posterior to the insertion of the rectus muscles and episcleritis is therefore anteriorly located.

Clinical features

Episcleritis is unilateral and frequently recurrent. It occurs more commonly in women and has a peak incidence between the ages of 30 and 40. The onset is sudden with intense redness, usually confined to one quadrant of the eye. A tender nodule may be present at the centre of the inflamed area and the patient complains of a pricking discomfort.

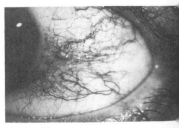

Episcleritis.

Causes

Frequently no underlying cause can be found but nodular episcleritis occurs in a variety of connective-tissue disorders including rheumatoid arthritis.

Management

Spontaneous remission occurs, usually within a few days. Topical steroids relieve discomfort and hasten resolution.

Scleritis

The sclera has a poor blood supply and, unlike the bright redness of episcleritis, inflammation of the sclera produces a dull purple-red patch.

Clinical features

A recurrent and not infrequently bilateral condition which can be extremely painful. It may be diffuse, nodular or necrotizing.

Causes

Scleritis is frequently associated with rheumatoid arthritis and occurs less commonly in a variety of other connective-tissue disorders such as Wegener's granulomatosis, polyarteritis nodosa and gout.

Nodular scleritis.

Management

Systemic steroids are the mainstay of treatment. Non-steroidal anti-inflammatory agents, such as oxyphenbutazone and indomethacin, may be effective in controlling the disease and immunosuppressives, such as cyclophosphamide and azathioprine, are used in combination with steroids.

Subconjunctival haemorrhage

Haemorrhage into the subconjunctival space may occur spontaneously in the middle aged and elderly, when it is often recurrent, or be caused by trauma. There is no significant association with systemic vascular disease.

The haemorrhage remains bright red until it begins to fade after a period of several days.

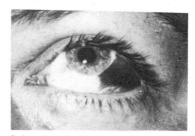

Subconjunctival haemorrhage.

The irritable eye   8

Many patients complain of sore, burning or itchy eyes. A consequence of the rich sensory innervation of the lids, conjunctiva and cornea is that superficial lesions of the eye can cause considerable discomfort, often out of proportion to the signs produced.

There are many causes of these symptoms but the more frequent include :

1. **Blepharitis**

   Chronic inflammation of the lid margins which causes an uncomfortable, burning sensation. The cause is usually chronic staphylococcal infection and there may be secondary involvement of the conjunctiva and cornea (*see* Chapter 12).

2. **Inturning lashes**

   Inturning lashes in trichiasis and entropion (*see* Chapter 12) irritate the cornea causing a persistent foreign body sensation.

3. **Chronic conjunctivitis**

   Chronic allergic conjunctivitis can cause symptoms ranging from slight pricking discomfort to intense irritation. A less common cause of persistent conjunctivitis is viral infection of the lid margin, for example by the molluscum and papovaviruses.

   Keratoconjunctivitis sicca (*see* Chapter 9) causes chronic ocular discomfort. In the milder forms the eyes may appear normal but special investigations reveal tear deficiency.

4. **Poor lid closure**

   This is usually the result of facial palsy or severe proptosis. The lower cornea becomes dry and ulcerated, particularly during sleep. Artificial tear drops, ointment and, occasionally, lateral tarsorrhaphy are required.

Non-specific ocular irritation

Many patients complain that their eyes are constantly sore and that the symptoms are aggravated by hot, dry and smoky conditions. Examination reveals either no abnormality or very mild conjunctival hyperaemia. The cause of this common complaint is poorly understood and symptomatic relief is only occasionally obtained by the use of artificial tear drops and conjunctival decongestants.

The dry eye 9

Tear deficiency produces a spectrum of disease ranging from minor discomfort to severe pain and blindness.

A stable tear film is essential for the maintenance of corneal clarity. It has important nutritional and protective functions and a deficiency of normal tears results in corneal and conjunctival damage.

The normal tear film consists of three layers :

1. *A thin layer of mucus*, derived from conjunctival goblet cells, which allows the aqueous tears to adhere to the cornea.

2. *Aqueous tears*, from the lacrimal gland, which contain immunoglobulins and the antibacterial protein, lysozyme.

3. *A superficial lipid layer*, derived from the secretions of the Meibomian glands, which retards evaporation of the aqueous tears.

Tears flow from the lacrimal gland to the lacrimal puncta mainly along the lower lid margin. The action of the upper lid is essential in applying mucus to the corneal surface and in ensuring an even spread of tears over the cornea.

Clinical features

Patients with dry eyes complain of chronic discomfort, usually described as a burning, gritty sensation. With minor degrees of tear deficiency signs may be minimal but more severe dryness is accompanied by conjunctival hyperaemia, reduced corneal lustre and the accumulation of stringy mucus.

Assessment of tear deficiency is carried out by :

1. Measurement of the rate of aqueous tear formation—*Schirmer's test*. Absorbent paper strips are placed with one end in the lower fornix. The length of paper wetted in 5 min is an indication of the rate of formation. Less than 10 mm suggests deficiency.

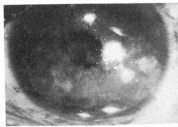
Dry eye—lack of corneal lustre.

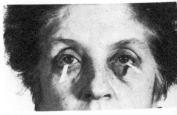
Schirmer's test.

2. Staining with *Rose Bengal*. Diseased conjunctival and corneal cells are stained by this dye and characteristic patterns are seen in dry eyes.

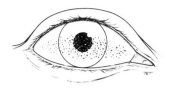

Staining of conjunctiva and cornea with Rose Bengal.

Causes

1. LACRIMAL GLAND DISEASE

Decreased lacrimal secretion (keratoconjunctivitis sicca) is often associated with rheumatoid arthritis, or another collagen disease, as part of Sjögren's syndrome (*see* Chapter 28) or may occur in other multisystem disorders, such as sarcoidosis.

2. CONJUNCTIVAL SCARRING

This results in the loss of mucus-secreting goblet cells and in severe cases the aqueous tears are also reduced by obstruction of the lacrimal secretory ducts which open into the upper conjunctival fornix. Conjunctival scarring may be caused by:

a. Trachoma (*see* Chapter 6).

b. Vitamin A deficiency (*see* Chapter 6).   - Bitot spots react to cornea.

c. Stevens Johnson syndrome in which ocular inflammation is associated with erythema multiforme, mucocutaneous ulceration and polyarthralgia (*see* Chapter 31).

d. Ocular pemphigoid, a disease of unknown aetiology in which there is progressive conjunctival scarring and the formation of adhesions between the bulbar and tarsal conjunctiva (symblepharon) (*see* Chapter 31).

e. Thermal and chemical injuries.

Management

1. Artificial tear drops which must be regularly and frequently instilled.

2. Occlusion of the lacrimal puncta to conserve the natural tears is occasionally helpful.

3. Topical antibiotics may be required to control or prevent secondary bacterial infection.

The watering eye   10

Persistent watering of the eye is uncomfortable and socially embarrassing. It may cause blurring of the vision and soreness of the skin at the inner and outer canthi.

Ocular irritation and emotional upset cause *lacrimation* with spillage of excess tears. Defects in the lacrimal drainage system cause *epiphora* and may lead to infection.

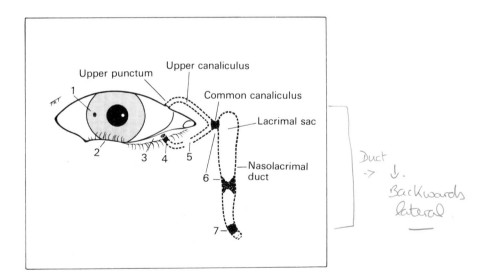

Causes

A. Lacrimation
1. *Corneal* foreign body, abrasion or inflammation.
2. *Entropion* or ingrowing eyelashes.

B. Epiphora

3. *Displacement* of the lower lid and *punctum* in ectropion and facial palsy (lagophthalmos) (*see* Chapter 12).

4. *Blocked punctum*. This is uncommon. It may be caused by chronic infection (staphylococcal or herpes simplex) or chronic drug administration (idoxuridine drops).

5. *Canalicular obstruction*. This may be due to chronic infection with staphylococcus or streptothrix or result from a laceration of the lids.

6. *Adult obstruction of the nasolacrimal duct*. Stenosis of the duct leads to stagnation of tears and eventual infection. The patient is troubled by epiphora which is often accompanied by varying amounts of mucopurulent discharge.

If the common canaliculus is obstructed as well a mucocele may develop. Infection in this situation leads to acute *dacryocystitis* with abscess formation. This presents as an exquisitely painful swelling pointing at the side of the nose just below the medial canthal ligament.

7. *Nasolacrimal duct obstruction in infants*. Incomplete canalization of the lower end of the duct is a common cause of the watering sticky eye in children under 6 months of age.

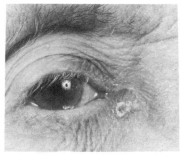

Acute dacryocystitis—abscess has discharged through skin.

Management

1,2,3 and 4 can be diagnosed by careful inspection and the cause removed or corrected surgically.

5 and 6 are diagnosed by probing and syringing of the lacrimal passages. The site of an obstruction can be further delineated by contrast radiology (dacryocystography). If symptoms merit treatment canalicular obstructions can be excised and nasolacrimal duct stenosis bypassed by dacryocystorhinostomy (DCR) (*see* Chapter 35). Acute dacryocystitis requires systemic antibiotic therapy and, when the infection has completely subsided, DCR.

7. Spontaneous cure by the age of 9 months is the rule and this may be aided by regular massage over the lacrimal sac. After this age probing of the nasolacrimal duct is carried out under general anaesthesia. Patency is confirmed by syringing.

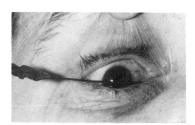

Probing of the nasolacrimal duct. a, probe in canaliculus and sac;

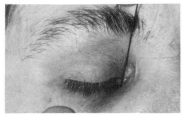

b, probe rotated and passed down into duct.

Headache and facial pain

It is important to be aware of the different patterns of headache and facial pain for the widespread distribution of the fifth cranial nerve means that these symptoms can originate from disorders of the eyes, sinuses, teeth, joints and central nervous system.

Ocular disease

Inflammatory disease and acute rises in intraocular pressure may cause pain in and around the eye and headache. However, the associated clinical features, such as loss of vision or redness, combined with an ophthalmic examination seldom leave doubt as to the cause. For example, the pain of *subacute glaucoma* is almost invariably accompanied by misting of the vision and frequently by rainbow haloes. Although the attack will usually have subsided by the time of examination this will reveal an abnormally narrow drainage angle.

'Eye strain'

Although this term is frequently used it is often difficult for the patient to describe the symptoms accurately. There is usually ocular discomfort with the lids feeling hot and swollen. Vision may be blurred, particularly during reading when the print appears to swim or become doubled. Frontal headache may also develop. However, the key feature of eye strain is that the symptoms are *related to visual effort*.

The eyes themselves appear normal but examination may reveal uncorrected refractive errors, accomodative fatigue, poor convergence or difficulty in controlling a latent squint (*see* Chapter 19).

The symptoms are often relieved by the prescription of appropriate spectacles or exercises but there is little justification for the incrimination and correction of minor refractive errors for non-specific headaches which are unrelated to visual effort.

Tension

The commonest cause of repeated and persistent headache is 'tension'. The headaches may last for days or even weeks on end and are described as being like constricting bands around the head or deep-seated pain behind the eyes. They are not relieved by simple analgesics. Some patients are consoled by the news that there is no ocular or intracranial disease but others visit a succession of different specialists whose investigations are invariably negative.

Intracranial headache

Behind the symptom of repeated headache often lurks the fear of a brain tumour. Raised intracranial pressure causes headache which is classically present on waking, intermittent, aggravated by straining and relieved by simple analgesics. The ocular examination of a patient presenting with this type of headache should be directed towards the detection of a cranial nerve palsy, papilloedema or visual field defect. In the absence of these and any other neurological abnormality most patients require reassurance only.

The headache of subarachnoid haemorrhage or meningitis is severe and a neurological cause is usually obvious.

Hypertension

Moderate hypertension seldom produces headache but acute accelerated hypertension can cause severe discomfort. The fundus changes of papilloedema, haemorrhages and exudates assist in making the diagnosis (see Chapter 26).

Migraine

The headache of classical migraine is frequently accompanied by visual phenomena including field loss (see Chapter 4). The diagnosis is made on the history and lack of abnormal findings.

Migrainous neuralgia

This variant of migraine causes severe pain in one eye which typically wakes the patient at night. The eye is often red and watering and the pain lasts for 2 or 3 hours. The attacks come in 'clusters' and after a period of a few weeks suddenly stop. Treatment consists of the prophylactic use of ergotamine tartrate.

Trigeminal neuralgia

The excruciating pain of trigeminal neuralgia (tic douloureux) has an abrupt onset and affects the eye, cheek and teeth on one side. The severity and distribution of the pain are diagnostic.

Herpes zoster ophthalmicus

Pain in the distribution of the first division of the trigeminal nerve precedes vesicle formation (*see* Chapter 29). Post-herpetic neuralgia may last for many months.

Giant-cell (temporal) arteritis

This is an uncommon cause of headache but should be considered in the elderly. The importance of making an early diagnosis lies in the possibility of preventing disastrous visual loss (*see* Chapter 28).

Referred pain

Pain may be referred to the eye from adjacent structures, particularly the sinuses and teeth, and this can give rise to diagnostic problems. Ocular pain may also result from more distant disease, such as cervical spondylosis.

Section 3

Abnormal appearance

The eyelids 12

Ptosis

Ptosis means drooping of the upper eyelid. It is most readily recognized when unilateral.

The palpebral apertures are normally symmetrical, the upper lid margin lying just above the pupil and the lower lid margin at the lower pole of the cornea.

The upper lid is elevated by the levator palpebrae superioris which is supplied by the third nerve and, to a small extent, by the sympathetically-innervated smooth muscle of Müller.

Congenital ptosis

This is caused by weakness of the levator muscle. It may be hereditary and either unilateral or bilateral. If the visual axis is covered the child may attempt to elevate the lid through overaction of the frontalis muscle or an abnormal head posture may be adopted with the chin elevated. If the visual axis cannot be cleared vision will fail to develop normally (sensory amblyopia) (*see* Chapter 19).

Surgical correction is indicated for visual or cosmetic reasons.

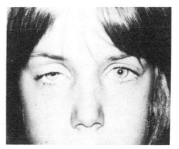

Congenital ptosis.

Acquired ptosis

Neurogenic
1. THIRD NERVE PALSY

The ptosis is often complete. There is defective ocular movement and usually the pupil is dilated.

2. HORNER'S SYNDROME

A small degree of ptosis accompanied by slight pupillary constriction is caused by interruption of the sympathetic nerve supply (*see* Chapter 27).

(from Hypothalamus to orbit)
Pg135.

③ - Loss of sweating over the forehead.

69

Myogenic

1. SENILE

This is due to <u>degenerative changes in the levator</u> and <u>its aponeurosis</u> and is the <u>commonest cause of ptosis</u>. Surgical correction is required if vision is affected.

2. MYASTHENIA GRAVIS

<u>Ptosis is often the first sign of this condition</u>. Typically it is <u>variable, asymmetrical</u> and <u>accompanied by diplopia</u> (*see* Chapter 27). *pg 134*

└due to ophthalmoplegia. (Rarely affects intrinsic Muscles of the eye!)

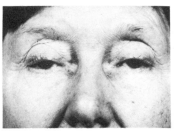

Senile ptosis.

Mechanical

Ptosis may result from any swelling of the upper lid, whether due to <u>inflammation</u>, a <u>tumour</u> or <u>vascular abnormality</u> and will <u>persist until the underlying cause has been corrected</u>.

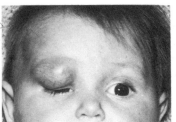

Mechanical ptosis due to haemangioma.

Other malpositions of the eyelids

Lid retraction

Lid retraction may be <u>unilateral or bilateral</u> and is almost invariably due to *thyroid disease*. The mechanism is not understood but sympathetic overactivity of Müller's muscle is thought to play a part.

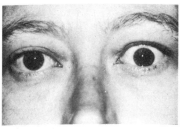

Lid retraction.

Lagophthalmos *c̄ Bells palsy!*

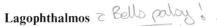

<u>Seventh nerve palsy</u> results in <u>incomplete closure of the eyelids</u>. The <u>lower lid falls away</u> from the globe and tears accumulate in the inferior conjunctival sac. If <u>Bell's phenomenon (elevation of the globe on attempted closure of the eyelids)</u> is intact the cornea may escape damage from exposure but lateral tarsorrhaphy (*see* Chapter 35) is required if ulceration of the lower cornea occurs.

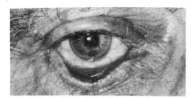

Lagophthalmos.

Entropion

Senile

<u>Laxity of the tissues allows the orbicularis muscle to tip the lower tarsal plate inwards causing inversion of the eyelid</u>. The lashes irritate the conjunctiva and cornea and <u>surgical correction</u> (*see* Chapter 35) is necessary.

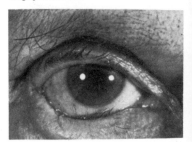

Senile entropion.

Cicatricial

This may involve the upper or lower eyelid. Trauma and trachoma are the commonest causes. Treatment is by surgical correction of the deformity and protection of the cornea by epilation of the offending lashes or the provision of a protective contact lens.

Ectropion

Senile

Eversion of the lower lid, due to laxity of the eyelid tissues, results in exposure of the tarsal conjunctiva and epiphora due to displacement of the lower lacrimal punctum. Treatment is surgical (*see* Chapter 35).

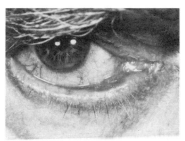

Senile ectropion.

Cicatricial

This may be caused by trauma, especially burns, or tumours involving the skin of the eyelids. Treatment is surgical but temporary measures to protect the cornea may be required.

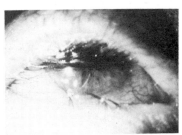

Trichiasis.

Trichiasis

Misalignment of the eyelashes is a consequence of scarring of the eyelids margin from infection or trauma. Treatment is required if the lashes abrade the cornea. Simple epilation gives temporary relief but permanent removal by electrolysis, cryosurgery or surgical transplantation of the lashes is necessary.

Abnormal movements of the eyelids

Blinking and closure of the eyelids are effected by the orbicularis oculi muscle innervated by the seventh nerve.

Blepharospasm

Forcible and repeated closure of the eyelids may be caused by any irritating lesion of the anterior segment of the eye. When chronic and without organic cause the condition is known as essential blepharospasm; permanent relief is difficult to obtain.

Myokymia

A fluttering of the eyelid which can be felt by the patient and seen on close inspection. This common condition is due to myoclonic movements of the orbicularis muscle. The cause is unknown but there is no serious underlying disease.

Inflammations

Blepharitis

A common, chronic relapsing inflammation of the eyelid margins. There is frequently staphylococcal infection with associated conjunctivitis or keratitis. The eyelid margins are red and scaly and in severe cases swollen and ulcerated. Treatment consists of lid bathing to remove the scales and application of antibiotic ointment. Topical steroids and systemic tetracycline are occasionally necessary to control the disease.

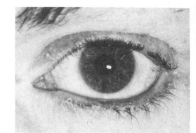

Squamous blepharitis.

Stye

A painful infection, usually staphylococcal, of a lash follicle. Treatment consists of local heat to encourage pointing and discharge of the abscess and the application of local antibiotic ointment. Systemic antibiotics are occasionally necessary if cellulitis of the lid develops. Surgical drainage, however, is seldom required.

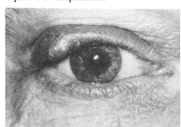

Stye.

Meibomian cyst

A retention cyst of the Meibomian gland which may become infected or develop into a chronic granuloma (chalazion). Treatment of an infected cyst is the same as for a stye. Non-infected cysts and chalazia are treated by incision and curettage (*see* Chapter 35).

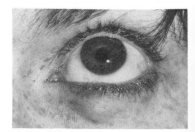

Meibomian cyst in lower lid.

Dacryoadenitis

Inflammation of the lacrimal gland results in pain and swelling of the outer part of the upper eyelids. Causes include mumps and sarcoidosis.

Herpes zoster ophthalmicus

Pain precedes the rash which erupts in the distribution of the first division of the trigeminal nerve. In severe

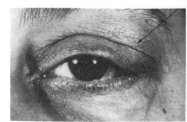

Dacryoadenitis.

Antiviral ; steroids !—TOPICAL. [handwritten annotation]

cases necrosis of the lids may occur. The eye itself may or may not be involved (*see* Chapter 29).

conjunctivitis - common ; keratitis - Mild - Ant Uveitis — 2° Glaucoma. punctate ulcers → Dendritic → Scarring [handwritten annotation]

Primary herpes simplex

This usually occurs in childhood producing clusters of vesicles around the eyelids. There is often an associated conjunctivitis. There may be pyrexia and systemic malaise (*see* Chapter 29).

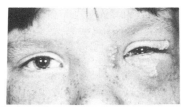

Primary herpes simplex.

Dermatitis

Contact dermatitis of the lids is usually due to topical medications, less frequently to cosmetics. Atropine, chloramphenicol and neomycin are common causes but preservatives in eyedrops may be responsible. The skin is red, swollen and intensely irritating. Treatment consists of identifying and removing the irritant.

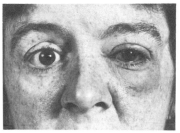

Contact dermatitis.

Tumours

Papillomas

These tumours are frequently pedunculated with a fibrovascular core. Treatment consists of excision with cautery to the base.

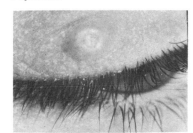

Papilloma.

Warts

Multilobulated lesions, often arising on the lid margin and caused by viruses of the papovavirus group. They may cause chronic conjunctivitis. Treatment consists of removal by curettage.

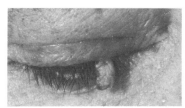

Molluscum contagiosum

These are small umbilicated lesions caused by the molluscum virus. If present close to the lid margin they cause conjunctivitis. Treatment consists of excision or curettage and chemical cautery.

Molluscum contagiosum.

Xanthelasmas

These creamy coloured lesions arising in the skin of the upper and lower lids close to the inner canthi are caused by lipid deposition within the dermis. They occur in hypercholesterolaemia; investigation of lipid metabolism is required. Excision is for cosmetic reasons only.

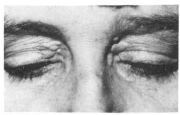

Xanthelasmas.

Marginal cysts

Clear cysts are derived from sweat glands (cysts of Moll); white cysts are derived from sebaceous glands (cysts of Zeis). Both are treated by excision.

Basal-cell carcinoma

This slowly progressive tumour, also known as a *rodent ulcer*, is common in exposed areas and frequently occurs in the region of the lower eyelid. Typically it has a rolled edge with a central area of ulceration which repeatedly forms a scab. The tumour spreads locally but very rarely metastasizes. Treatment is by surgical excision, radiotherapy or cryotherapy, depending on the precise location and size of the tumour.

Squamous-cell carcinoma

An uncommon tumour around the eyelids. Some are similar in appearance to a basal-cell carcinoma, others may be mistaken for inflammatory lesions. Untreated, a squamous-cell carcinoma causes severe ulceration and may metastasize. Treatment is by excision.

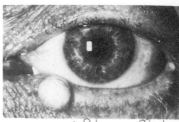

Cyst of Zeis. ⇒ Sebaceous Gland.

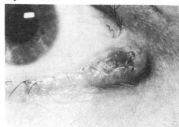

Basal-cell carcinoma.

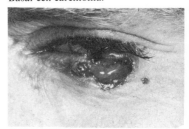

Squamous-cell carcinoma.

Proptosis

13

(handwritten notes)

1. Thyroid eye disease
2. Lymphoma
3. Sinusitis   esp ethmoidal.
4. Optic N. Glioma ⎤
5. Rhabdomyosarcoma ⎦
6. Pseudo-tumour of Orbit = Granulomatous Rxn.

7. caratico cavernous fistula
8. Haematoma of orbit.
9. Cellulitis " "

Proptosis means forward protrusion of the eye and lids and is virtually synonymous with the term '*exophthalmos*' which implies forward protrusion of the eye alone. As the orbital tissues are surrounded by bone any increase in their content will push the globe forward.

The degree of proptosis may be assessed by inspection or with an exophthalmometer which measures the distance between the outer angle of the orbit and the corneal apex.

Plain x-ray and computerized tomography (CT scan) are the principal investigations of orbital disease.

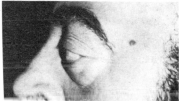

Proptosis.

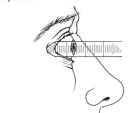

Exophthalmometry.

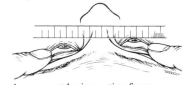

Assessment by inspection from above.

Dysthyroid eye disease

This is the commonest cause of both unilateral and bilateral proptosis. It is caused mainly by swelling of the extraocular muscles and lymphocytic infiltration of the orbital tissues (*see* Chapter 25).

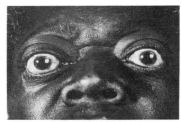

Thyroid exophthalmos.

Tumour of the orbit

Clinical features

These uncommon tumours present as unilateral proptosis. Tumours arising within the cone of the extraocular muscles cause axial proptosis and visual loss while tumours outside the muscle cone tend to cause additional vertical or horizontal displacement of the globe, often resulting in diplopia. Most tumours of the orbit are primary. Secondary deposits are uncommon.

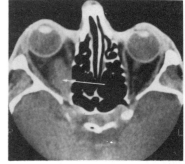

CT scan of intraconal tumour, causing proptosis.

Causes

Those arising within the muscle cone include:
1. Optic nerve glioma
2. Optic nerve meningioma
3. Haemangioma
4. Orbital varices

Those arising outside the muscle cone include:
1. Lymphoma
2. Mixed cell tumour of the lacrimal gland
3. Extension of tumours from the nasopharynx

Orbital tumours in childhood include:
1. Rhabdomyosarcoma
2. Neuroblastoma from the adrenals

Management

The investigation of an orbital tumour is essentially radiological but the diagnosis may be confirmed by biopsy where appropriate. Treatment, when indicated, is by surgical excision or radiotherapy.

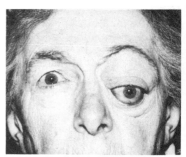

Mixed cell tumour of the lacrimal gland.

Orbital pseudotumour

This condition is caused by a granulomatous reaction to a variety of diseases. The proptosis is usually accompanied by pain or discomfort and limitation of eye movements causes diplopia. The diagnosis is made from radiological studies or biopsy. Treatment is with systemic steroids or radiotherapy.

Orbital cellulitis

Clinical features

The eye is proptosed and both the lids and conjunctiva are inflamed and swollen. Eye movements are limited and painful and there is frequently general malaise and fever.

Causes

Orbital cellulitis is usually the result of infection in a neighbouring sinus, the ethmoid and the frontal sinuses being the most commonly involved. Less commonly infection may be blood borne or introduced by trauma.

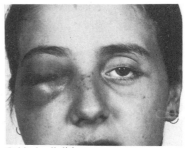
Orbital cellulitis.

Management

The underlying cause is usually diagnosed by x-ray of the sinuses. Treatment is essentially with systemic antibiotics but drainage of infected sinuses should be carried out by an ENT surgeon. Occasionally the formation of a subperiosteal orbital abscess or intense intraorbital pressure causes sudden irreversible loss of vision by obstruction of the optic nerve or retinal blood supply.

Cavernous sinus thrombosis

This rare but very serious condition may follow orbital cellulitis or other infection in the territory of the orbital veins. The clinical signs are similar to orbital cellulitis but usually both eyes are involved and vision is significantly diminished. The patient is gravely ill and mortality is high in spite of treatment.

Orbital haematoma

Clinical features

In addition to proptosis there is swelling and bruising of the lids, subconjunctival haemorrhage and limitation of ocular movement. Visual failure may result from the effects of increased orbital pressure.

Causes

Bleeding within the orbit is usually a result of severe head injury though it may occasionally occur in the elderly as a spontaneous event following a bout of coughing or straining. It is a potential complication of cosmetic lid surgery.

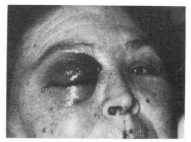
Orbital haematoma.

Management

If sight is threatened the haematoma may be evacuated via an anterior approach through the conjunctiva but this is seldom successful in restoring vision which is already lost.

Carotico-cavernous fistula

Clinical features

There is dramatic proptosis, of sudden onset, which may affect one or both eyes. In the early stages the conjunctiva is grossly oedematous and congested and the eye may pulsate in time with the arterial pulse. Later, when the oedema has resolved the surface veins remain dilated and are a prominent feature. There is a marked *bruit* audible to both patient and, with the aid of a stethoscope, observer. The vision may be seriously diminished as the high pressure within the ophthalmic veins (seen as papilloedema and venous congestion) may prevent adequate perfusion of the eye.

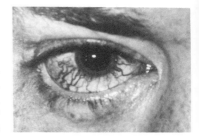

Carotico-cavernous fistula—dilated surface vessels.

Causes

The clinical signs are produced by the development of an arteriovenous fistula between the internal carotid artery and cavernous sinus. Trauma is a frequent cause but the condition may occur spontaneously, particularly in women.

Management

The fistula may close spontaneously or may be closed surgically by the introduction of a balloon catheter. The main indications for closure of a fistula are to halt advancing proptosis and eliminate the bruit which may make life intolerable for the patient.

Pseudoproptosis

Unilateral high myopia may be mistaken for proptosis. The affected eye is larger than the normal eye and protrudes further forward from the orbit. The degree of refractive error is usually over 10 dioptres and the vision seldom corrects completely to normal. The patient is usually aware that the vision has always been poor in this eye. It is important to recognize the condition and to avoid subjecting the patient to unnecessary investigations.

The conjunctiva, sclera and cornea

14

A wide variety of non-inflammatory conditions affect the anterior segment of the eye. Some are of little pathological significance but cause concern to the patient. Others may indicate serious ocular disease or reflect disease elsewhere in the body.

Conjunctiva

Pingueculae

These are small yellow nodules which appear on either side of the cornea within the palpebral fissure. They are very common in adults and are composed of hyaline and degenerative elastic tissue. They occasionally become inflamed but treatment is seldom required.

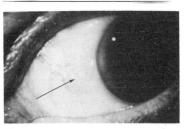

Pinguecula.

Pterygium

This is a fleshy growth of the conjunctiva across the cornea on the nasal side. Pterygia are very common in adults living in hot, sunny climates. Surgical removal (with postoperative beta-irradiation) is indicated for cosmetic reasons or if the pterygium approaches the visual axis. Recurrence following surgery is common.

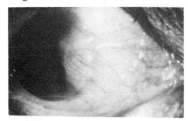

Pterygium.

Conjunctival cysts

These moderately common, small, translucent cysts are due to dilated lymphatic channels. Puncturing of the cyst or surgical excision is occasionally required.

Conjunctival naevi

Common in adolescents, these para-limbal lesions often become pigmented at the time of puberty. There is no significant malignant potential.

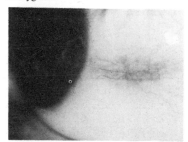

Conjunctival naevus.

79

Conjunctival melanosis

Pigmentation of the conjunctiva is common in the dark skinned races. The brown patches, usually near the limbus, have a very low malignant potential, and no treatment is required.

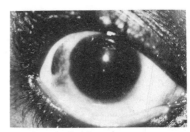

Conjunctival melanosis.

Malignant melanoma

This is uncommon. Clinically, a melanoma presents as a progressively enlarging shiny black/brown lesion. Surgical treatment varies from local excision to complete removal of the orbital contents (exenteration).

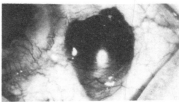

Jaundice

In obstructive jaundice bile pigments accumulate in the conjunctiva giving rise to the typical yellow appearance of the eyes.

Malignant melonoma of the conjunctiva.

Argyrosis

Slate-grey pigmentation of the conjunctiva follows prolonged use of silver nitrate drops, originally used as a prophylaxis against gonococcal ophthalmia neonatorum (*see* Chapter 29).

Sclera

Blue sclerae

A rare, bilateral, hereditary condition in which the sclera appears uniformly slate-grey or blue. This is due to thinning of the sclera which allows the uveal tissues to show through. This condition is frequently associated with bone fragility (osteogenesis imperfecta) and deafness due to otosclerosis.

Cornea

Arcus senilis

A very common, bilateral corneal condition. A ring of lipid is deposited in the peripheral cornea leaving a clear zone between arcus and limbus. Arcus senilis does not affect vision and is of little significance in the elderly. Lipid studies are merited in young patients. No treatment is required unless a significant abnormality of lipid metabolism is detected.

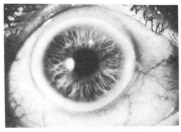

Arcus senilis.

Band degeneration *(Keratopathy).*

Calcium is deposited in the superficial cornea in a horizontal band. Causes include hypercalcaemia and chronic ocular inflammation (for example Still's disease) but in many cases no cause can be found. Treatment is required to relieve discomfort or if vision is affected. The calcium can be removed with the aid of a chelating agent, such as EDTA, which is applied directly to the cornea.

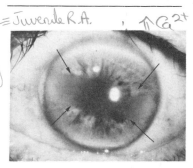

= Juvenile R.A. , ↑ Ca^{2+}

Band degeneration of the cornea.

Corneal dystrophies

These uncommon bilateral hereditary conditions cause corneal opacification and irregularity but without the neovascularization seen following keratitis. Treatment, for visual reasons, is by corneal grafting (*see* Chapter 35).

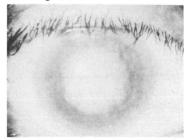

Corneal dystrophy — pupil obscured.

Kayser–Fleischer rings

Faint brown rings of copper deposited deep in the peripheral cornea. Vision is not affected. The rings occur in Wilson's disease and slit-lamp examination of the eyes may be the key to the correct diagnosis of this potentially fatal condition.

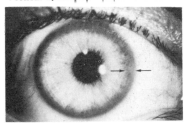

Kayser–Fleischer ring.

The pupil and iris 15

The iris consists of an anterior stroma of collagen fibres, chromatophores and blood vessels lying upon a layer of pigment epithelium. The sphincter muscle, with its parasympathetic innervation from the third nerve lies within the stroma near the pupil margin. The sympathetically-innervated dilator muscle is deep to the stroma.

Examination

The iris should be inspected with the aid of a focused torch for abnormalities of colour or movement and the shape and position of the pupil.

Pupillary reflexes

A bright light shone into one eye produces constriction of the pupil (*direct light reflex*) and a similar amount of constriction of the fellow pupil (*consensual light reflex*).

Constriction of the pupil also occurs during convergence (*near reaction*).

A lesion of the visual pathway anterior to the chiasm on one side only results in a *relative afferent pupillary defect*. The pupils are of equal size but when the normal side is covered the affected pupil, freed from its consensual reaction, dilates.

Corectopia => Pupil located acentrally

Pupils of abnormal shape

Congenital

Coloboma

A sector defect of the iris, usually inferonasal, caused by incomplete closure of the fetal ocular cleft. There may be an associated coloboma of the choroid or optic nerve with reduced vision.

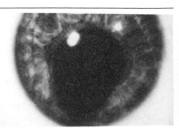
Coloboma of the iris.

Trauma → Iridodialysis , iris prolapse.

Acquired

Adhesions

The iris may develop synechiae anteriorly to the cornea or posteriorly to the lens as a result of inflammatory disease or trauma. The abnormal shape may only be apparent when the pupil is dilated. *NB*

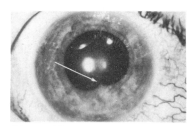
Iris synechia.

Surgical defects

Iridectomies, both peripheral and sector, are usually performed superiorly so that the defect is covered by the lid.

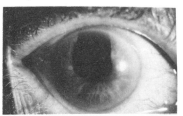
Sector iridectomy.

Tumour

Malignant tumours of the iris cause increasing irregularity of the pupil as they enlarge.

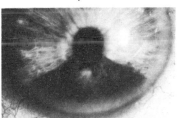
Malignant melanoma of the iris.

Pupils of abnormal size

Unequal pupils—anisocoria

A small inequality of pupil size occurs in about 20% of normal people; the pupil reflexes are normal.

1. THIRD NERVE PALSY

The affected pupil is about two-thirds dilated and does not react to light or near stimulus.

fixed + Dilated

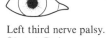
Left third nerve palsy.

2. HORNER'S SYNDROME *Miosis, ptosis, anhydrosis} -on affected side .*

The affected pupil is smaller than the normal side and is due to a lesion affecting the sympathetic nerve supply to the dilator muscle. The pupil inequality is best seen in dim light.

Left Horner's syndrome.

3. TONIC PUPIL (HOLMES–ADIE SYNDROME)

The affected pupil is dilated and reacts very slowly to light and to a near stimulus. Eventually, both pupils may be involved. The condition affects mainly young

Left Holmes–Adie pupil.

ɣ women. Deep tendon reflexes affecting the knees and ankles are absent and it is thought that the syndrome is due to a disorder of the sensory ganglia. The pupil shows a supersensitivity to weak cholinergic drops.

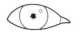 ? Viral infection.

4. ARGYLL ROBERTSON PUPILS

The pupils are small, unequal in size and irregular. They do not react to light though they do constrict on accommodation (light-near dissociation). These features are characteristic of *neurosyphilis*.

Argyll Robertson pupils.

5. POST-TRAUMATIC

A contusion injury may damage the sphincter muscle causing permanent dilatation of the pupil which gives rise to discomfort and dazzle in bright light.

Loss of accommodation

6. IRIS ISCHAEMIA

Ischaemic damage to the iris may occur in acute glaucoma and herpes zoster ophthalmicus resulting in an enlarged, often irregular pupil.

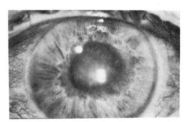

Iris ischaemia following herpes zoster.

Small pupils—miosis

The pupils are constricted with poor or absent dilatation in the dark. Causes include:
1. Old age (senile miosis).
2. Drugs: (*a*) Pilocarpine drops used in the treatment of chronic glaucoma. (*b*) Morphine and related drugs.

Large pupils—mydriasis

The pupils are dilated and fail to constrict to a light. Causes include:
1. Topical atropine or atropine-like drugs. The pupil fails to respond to pilocarpine in contrast to the dilatation of a third nerve lesion.
2. Bilateral blindness due to lesions anterior to the lateral geniculate bodies. The pupils do not react to light but respond briskly to pilocarpine drops.

Pupil reactions in the unconscious patient

Examination of the pupil reactions in the unconscious patient provides a guide to brainstem function.
1. If a patient develops a dilated and non-reacting pupil on one side this indicates third nerve involvement from brainstem compression or distortion, e.g. from herniation of the cerebral hemisphere through the tentorium. If both pupils become affected the general state of the patient is grave.

2. If both pupils are miosed this indicates a pontine lesion.

The abnormal iris

The colour of the iris is determined by the amount of pigment in the stroma.

Heterochromia

A difference in colour between the two eyes may be congenital or due to :
1. Chronic, severe inflammatory disease of one eye.
2. Iris tumour.
3. Heterochromic cyclitis—a disease of unknown origin in which the lighter coloured eye suffers from a low-grade anterior uveitis and frequently develops cataract and glaucoma.
4. Siderosis. A retained ferrous intraocular foreign body results in the widespread distribution of iron in the ocular tissues. Anterior segment involvement results in darkening of the iris and secondary glaucoma.

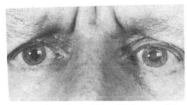

Heterochromic cyclitis of left eye with cataract.

Neovascularization

New vessel growth on the surface of the iris (rubeosis iridis) occurs in the eye with an ischaemic retina. This is most commonly seen in patients with *proliferative diabetic retinopathy* and following *central retinal vein occlusion*. The new vessels may occasionally be visible to the naked eye but a more prominent feature is eversion of the pupil margin (ectropion uvea) caused by contraction of the fibrovascular membrane on the surface of the iris. The drainage angle of the eye is obliterated, resulting in intractable 'thrombotic' glaucoma.

Albinism

An uncommon, bilateral hereditary condition. When severe it is associated with macular hypoplasia causing diminished vision, photophobia, nystagmus and squint. Lack of pigment in the uveal tract causes the pupil to appear red. The skin, hair, eyebrows and lashes may be devoid of pigment. High refractive errors are common and tinted lenses are prescribed.

Iridodonesis

If the lens has been removed or is dislocated the iris loses its support and becomes tremulous.

The vitreous and fundus

16

Ophthalmoscopy during routine clinical examination or sight testing for spectacles may reveal an abnormal appearance in the asymptomatic patient. The pathologically cupped optic disc of chronic glaucoma is often the first sign of this serious disease but other fundus abnormalities, often provoking alarm, do not require further investigation if their nature is appreciated.

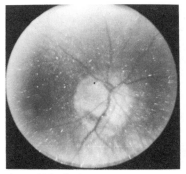

Asteroid hyalosis.

Asteroid hyalosis

White, spherical opacities are seen suspended in the vitreous which occasionally give rise to the symptom of floating spots. Eyes with this condition are essentially healthy though it is more common in diabetics.

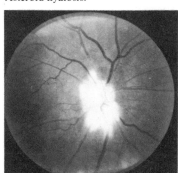

Myelinated fibres.

Myelinated nerve fibres

A fairly common congenital abnormality in which myelination of retinal nerve fibres gives rise to white patches, usually at the disc margin. The patches have a 'feathered' appearance and may partially obscure the retinal blood vessels. Vision is rarely affected to a significant degree but the abnormality may be mistaken for optic atrophy.

Colloid bodies  =Drusen

These hyaline bodies are the result of degenerative changes in Bruch's membrane which separates retina from choroid. They are most numerous in the macular area and may be mistaken for exudates. An increased risk of macular degeneration exists but treatment of the colloid bodies is not possible.

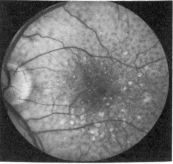

Colloid bodies.

Angioid streaks

This is an uncommon condition in which breaks in Bruch's membrane resemble blood vessels. Angioid streaks are associated with pseudoxanthoma elasticum and also occur, though less commonly, in Paget's disease and sickle-cell disease. They may give rise to disciform degeneration of the macula (*see* Chapter 3).

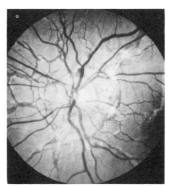

Angioid streaks.

Coloboma

An uncommon condition due to failure of closure of the fetal cleft. A large choroidal defect, usually below and extending up to the optic nerve, results in visual loss varying from minimal to severe. There may be an associated iris coloboma.

Choroidal naevi

Small, flat, pigmented choroidal lesions are common. The potential for malignant change is extremely small and no action is required.

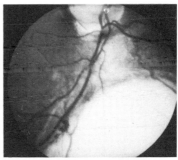

Coloboma of the fundus.

Tortuous retinal vessels

Unusual tortuosity of the retinal vessels may occur as a congenital abnormality. If the calibre of the vessels is normal and there are no haemorrhages the tortuosity is very unlikely to be of pathological significance.

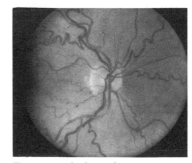

Tortuous retinal vessels.

Section 4

Abnormal eye movements,
double vision and squint

Eye movement and binocular single vision

17

The horizontal separation of the two eyes results in a slightly different image being formed on each retina. The fusion of these two images by higher centres in the brain allows *binocular single vision* with depth perception (stereopsis). Eye movements, initiated either visually from the occipital cortex, or voluntarily from the frontal cortex, are designed to direct both eyes at a given object and maintain binocular single vision.

Conjugate gaze

For distant objects the visual axes are virtually parallel and the movement of the two eyes in unison is called *conjugate gaze*. This is achieved by impulses from the higher centres of the brain being channelled through the medial longitudinal bundle which links the brain-stem nuclei associated with ocular movement. Thus conjugate gaze to the left side is mediated by the left sixth nerve innervating the left lateral rectus muscle and the right third nerve innervating the right medial rectus muscle.

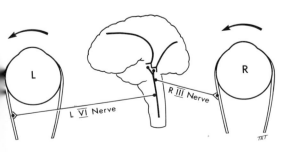

Left conjugate gaze.

Lesions above the nuclei (supranuclear) cause failure of conjugate movement (*gaze palsy*). The visual axes, however, remain parallel and double vision is not experienced.

For near objects the two eyes *converge*. This non-conjugate movement is mediated by the right and left third nerves innervating the medial recti muscles and is accompanied by accommodation of the lens and constriction of the pupils. Failure of convergence may cause double vision when regarding a near object.

Paralytic squint

Lesions at the level of the brainstem nuclei and below (infranuclear) result in misalignment of the visual axes due to limitation of movement in the direction of action of the affected muscle or groups of muscles. This is referred to as a *paralytic squint*. If this occurs once binocular single vision has fully developed *double vision* is experienced.

Concomitant squint   ⊊ Non Paralytic Squint!

In early childhood the causes and consequences of misalignment of the visual axes are quite different. Double vision does not occur and the squint is recognized only by the abnormal position of one eye. The ocular movements are usually full and the squint is present in all positions of gaze. This is referred to as a *concomitant squint*.

Nystagmus

Steadiness of the eyes during fixation of an object and smoothness of following movements are the result of complex feedback mechanisms involving the cerebral cortex, vestibular apparatus and cerebellum. Failure of these mechanisms causes *nystagmus*, an oscillatory movement of the eyes which is characteristically rhythmical. This may indicate serious ocular or neurological disease.

Paralytic squint and double vision

18

The main complaint of a patient presenting with a paralytic squint is double vision (diplopia) though the abnormal position of one eye in certain positions of gaze may be readily apparent to an independent observer.

Double vision caused by a paralytic squint (*binocular* diplopia) must be distinguished from *monocular* diplopia and *physiological* diplopia.

Monocular diplopia

In this condition double vision persists after the covering of one eye. There is only slight separation of the images, often described as 'ghosting'. The commonest causes are cataract and corneal scarring.

Physiological diplopia

When the eyes fixate a given point objects in front and behind this point appear double. However, this physiological diplopia is suppressed centrally and seldom reaches consciousness. Occasionally it is 'discovered' by a child who may be referred for investigation of double vision. It is diagnosed by the absence of defective eye movement and confirmed by demonstrating the nature of the double vision.

Binocular diplopia

In binocular diplopia the separation of the two images is maximal when the gaze is in the direction of the defective movement.

The ocular movements should be examined in the six cardinal positions of gaze to determine the direction in which the diplopia is greatest. In each position one muscle of each eye is predominantly acting. For example, if the separation of images is maximal on looking to the right either the right lateral rectus or left medial rectus muscle is at fault. Each eye is then covered in turn; the fainter and more peripheral image ✗ disappears on covering the *affected* eye.

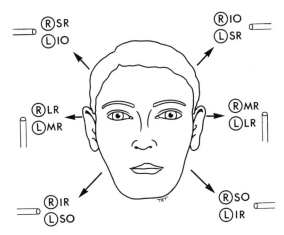

Ocular movements.

$LR_6(SO_4)$

Causes

Binocular diplopia may be caused by a nerve lesion, extraocular muscle disease or mechanical limitation of movement.

1. *Neurogenic.* A true paralytic squint is neurogenic. The nerve, or nerves, involved can be deduced from the pattern of defective eye movement.

a. Third nerve palsy. The superior, inferior and medial recti and inferior oblique muscles are affected and double vision is present in all positions of gaze other than lateral. Associated ptosis frequently eliminates the symptom of double vision. The pupil is often, though not invariably, dilated and unresponsive to light.

b. Fourth nerve palsy. Paralysis of the superior oblique muscle causes vertical separation of the images, maximal on looking down and in.

c. Sixth nerve palsy. Paralysis of the lateral rectus muscle causes horizontal diplopia maximal on looking to the side of the lesion.   · DM/MS/H Zoster/Trauma

d. Brainstem disease. Occlusive vertebrobasilar disease may cause transient diplopia due to involvement of the brainstem ocular motor nuclei.

eye looks ↓+out!
DM/H. Zoster/Aneurysm.

Vasc/H Zoster/Trauma

III

IV

VI

Vasc.
MS.

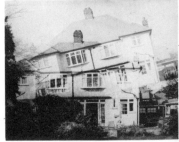

Binocular diplopia with vertical separation of the images.

Involvement of the medial longitudinal bundle, by vascular or demyelinating disease, causes internuclear ophthalmoplegia with double vision on lateral gaze (*see* Chapter 27).

2. *Muscular*

a. Myasthenia gravis. The double vision is variable and usually accompanied by ptosis.
b. Dysthyroid myopathy. The medial and inferior recti are most frequently involved.

3. *Mechanical*

a. Displacement of the globe by an orbital tumour.
b. Entrapment of orbital tissues in a 'blow-out' fracture (*see* Chapter 22).

Management

Once a true paralytic squint has been diagnosed the underlying cause must be sought. This requires a full medical examination to exclude diseases such as hypertension and diabetes, and neurological investigations to exclude an intracranial lesion.

The majority of non-traumatic paralytic squints improve either spontaneously or when the underlying disease is treated. Progress of resolution, which may take weeks or months, can be recorded on sequential Hess charts. This test records the separation of images in all positions of gaze.

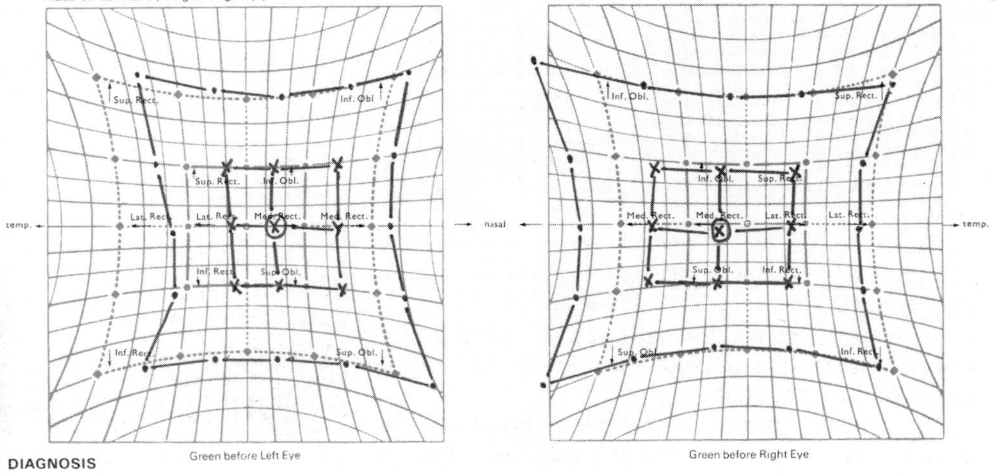

(handwritten margin notes:)
Co-ordination of Gaze of
CN III + VI is lost.
∴ → DV on Lat Gaze.

Pg 134.

Pg 121.

Causes
1 Vascular — DM, ↑BP, aterosclerosis Emboli
2. Inflammatory — MS. Sinusitis Meningitis Orbital Cellulitis H Zoster Syphilis
3 Neoplastic — Meningioma. astrocytoma Metastasis
4. Trauma
5. Aneurysm
6 Myasthenia Gravis / Myopathy 7

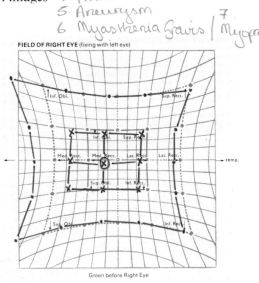

HESS SCREEN CHART
FIELD OF LEFT EYE (fixing with right eye) FIELD OF RIGHT EYE (fixing with left eye)

Sup. Rect. Inf. Obl.   Inf. Obl. Sup. Rect.
Sup. Rect. Inf. Obl.   Inf. Obl. Sup. Rect.
temp. Lat. Rect. Lat. Rect. Med Rect. Med. Rect. → nasal ← Med. Rect. Med. Rect. Lat. Rect. Lat. Rect. temp.
Inf. Rect. Sup. Obl.   Sup. Obl. Inf. Rect.
Inf. Rect. Sup. Obl.   Sup. Obl. Inf. Rect.

DIAGNOSIS   Green before Left Eye   Green before Right Eye

Hess chart of left sixth nerve palsy.

Relief of double vision may be obtained by :
1. Occlusion of one eye.
2. The incorporation of prisms into spectacles.
3. Muscle surgery when the paralytic squint shows no further sign of spontaneous improvement.

Concomitant squint 19

A squint in childhood is often first recognized or suspected by the parents when one eye appears to drift inwards or outwards. The majority of childhood squints are convergent (esotropia) and present before the age of 4; some are present at birth. Divergent squints (exotropia) tend to develop a little later.

Double vision is seldom appreciated by the young child because the image from the squinting eye is rapidly suppressed by the brain. This *suppression* interferes with the normal development of vision resulting in an *amblyopic* (lazy) eye.

Any suspected squint must be referred for ophthalmological assessment. *Amblyopia* is a serious but treatable condition.

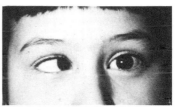

Right convergent squint.

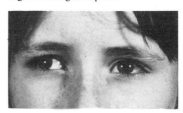

Right divergent squint.

Causes

1. *Genetic.* In most squints there is a failure of the central mechanism governing the development and maintenance of binocular single vision. This failure may be hereditary and is also commonly found where brain damage or mental retardation (e.g. Down's syndrome) exist.

2. *Refractive errors.* In emmetropic eyes the relationship between accommodation and convergence is balanced but in hypermetropia the extra accommodation required to produce a clear image on the retina may lead to excessive convergence and the development of a squint.

Accommodative Esotropia

3. *Ocular.* Ocular abnormalities, for example congenital cataract and retinoblastoma, may impair central vision in one or both eyes and prevent the fusion of images and the development of binocular vision.

Diagnosis

The appearance of a convergent squint in infants is often caused by broad epicanthic folds but a true squint can be detected by:

1. Inspection of the *corneal reflexes* with a torch light. These are normally symmetrical.
2. The *cover test*. If the eye fixating an object, such as a small toy, is covered, the squinting eye will move to take up fixation.

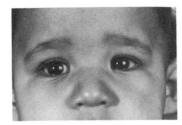

Apparent convergent squint due to epicanthic folds.

Management

The initial steps in the management of a squint are :

1. The assessment of *visual acuity* in each eye. In very young children an approximation of acuity can be obtained by observing the child's ability to pick up very small objects or follow an oscillating target (the Catford Drum).
2. *Ophthalmoscopy* to exclude ocular disease.
3. *Retinoscopy* to determine the presence of any significant refractive error.

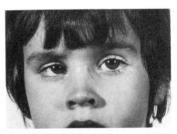

The Catford Drum.

Fundus examination and refraction are facilitated by the use of atropine drops or ointment in young children.

Subsequent steps are :

4. The *provision of glasses*, where appropriate, in order to improve visual acuity or restore a normal balance between accommodation and convergence. In some squints binocular vision can be restored by correcting the associated hypermetropia. These are known as *accommodative* squints.
5. If the vision in the squinting eye is defective and cannot be corrected simply by the provision of glasses amblyopia is present. *Occlusion* of the fellow eye forces use of the amblyopic eye and encourages the development of normal visual acuity. Occlusion is most successful when carried out soon after the development of a squint. Little benefit is obtained from occlusion after the age of eight, by which time development of vision is normally complete.
6. *Squint surgery* (*see* Chapter 35) is carried out to reduce the angle of squint. Restoration of *full binocular single vision is relatively uncommon* with convergent squints and surgery is usually cosmetic. Ideally it is carried out when amblyopia has been treated and when vision and fixation are equal in both eyes (*alternating convergent squint*).

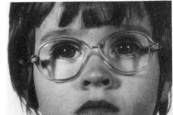

Accommodative squint (*a*) corrected by glasses (*b*).

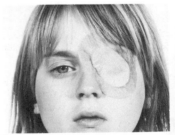

Occlusion.

The less common divergent squint is frequently intermittent and binocular vision continues to develop normally. Surgery is delayed until the increasing divergence of the eyes causes symptoms.

Latent squint

Few people have perfect ocular muscle balance. Most have some degree of latent squint but the potential deviation of the eyes is held in check by the power of fusion, preventing double vision. The commonest form is latent divergence (exophoria) followed by latent convergence (esophoria) and less commonly vertical deviation. Any generalized debility or illness may lead to decompensation of a latent squint resulting in a manifest squint. A latent squint that is controlled only with difficulty may cause eyestrain. Symptomatic relief may be obtained by the incorporation of prisms into glasses but squint surgery is often necessary.

Orthoptists

In the United Kingdom much of the diagnosis and management of patients with squint is carried out by orthoptists who are specially trained to deal with abnormalities of binocular vision and eye movement.

Nystagmus

20

Nystagmus is readily recognized as an abnormal oscillatory movement of the eyes. The pattern of the movement is broadly determined by the underlying disorder which may be congenital or acquired.

Congenital nystagmus

Pendular

The to and fro movements of the eyes are of equal velocity and give rise to a searching appearance. This type of nystagmus results from poor vision and is common in eyes with severe congenital developmental defects.

Jerk

This type of nystagmus is caused by a genetic defect in the ocular tracking mechanism and is often hereditary. The movements are jerky with a fast component toward the side of gaze. The eyes themselves are clinically normal but examination of the fundi may be difficult. There is usually a position of gaze in which the nystagmus is least marked (the null point) and children may adopt an abnormal head posture in order to achieve this. Distance vision is usually reduced to 6/18 or worse but reading vision is relatively good as the nystagmus is reduced on convergence.

Latent

In this condition, if both eyes are open fixation is steady and vision is normal but if one eye is covered the other develops a jerky nystagmus with reduction in visual acuity. This is usually discovered during routine testing of visual acuity and is often associated with a squint.

Acquired nystagmus

Gaze nystagmus

Nystagmus is often seen in normal individuals if the eyes are kept at the extreme of lateral gaze for more than a short period of time. This 'end point' nystagmus is due to fatigue and is of no significance.

True *gaze paretic nystagmus* is the most minor form of a gaze palsy. The lesion is supranuclear and may be caused by vascular, demyelinating or neoplastic lesions or by drug toxicity. The nystagmus is absent on forward gaze but occurs on deviation of the eyes with the fast component of the nystagmus being in the direction of gaze.

Vestibular nystagmus

Disease of the labyrinth and eighth nerve causes horizontal jerk nystagmus, often with a rotary element, toward the side opposite the lesion. There is always an associated acoustic disturbance.

Central vestibular nystagmus, caused by brainstem and cerebellar disease, may be horizontal, vertical or rotary but the direction of the fast phase does not indicate the side of the lesion.

Vestibular nystagmus is faster than gaze nystagmus. It can be simulated by rotation and caloric stimulation of the labyrinth.

Rare forms of nystagmus may have particular localizing value. These include:

See-saw nystagmus

One eye elevates and rotates inwards while the other depresses and rotates outwards. It is pathognomonic of a chiasmal lesion and there is almost invariably a complete bitemporal hemianopia.

Retractory nystagmus

Lesions affecting the region of the upper colliculi (e.g. pinealoma) cause failure of upward conjugate gaze associated with beats of nystagmus which retract the eyes into the orbit. It is associated with an abnormality of pupil reaction with poor response to light but normal near reaction (light-near dissociation).

Up-beat nystagmus

This is jerk nystagmus of large amplitude. The fast phase increases on upgaze and decreases on downgaze. It may be drug induced but is usually due to cerebellar disease.

Down-beat nystagmus

Characteristically caused by compressive lesions at the level of foramen magnum.

Optokinetic nystagmus

This is a physiological type of fixation nystagmus initated by movements of the environment and readily seen in an individual gazing out of the side of a moving vehicle ('railway' nystagmus). Clinically it can be induced with a rotating striped drum. In patients with homonymous hemianopia due to lesions of the parietal cortex optokinetic nystagmus is usually abolished.

The demonstration of optokinetic nystagmus is a useful test for the malingerer who claims blindness in one or both eyes. Presented with the rotating drum he is unable to prevent the induced nystagmus.

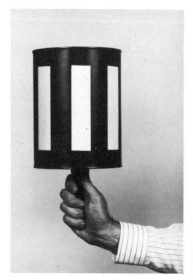

Optokinetic drum.

Section 5

Trauma

Minor trauma

21

The eye is well protected by rapid reflex closure of the eyelids yet trauma to the cornea is commonplace. This is usually minor in the sense that recovery is rapid and without serious consequence but to the patient it may be extremely painful and, without proper treatment, can result in disastrous loss of vision.

Corneal foreign body

Clinical features

In common with other forms of corneal trauma the eye is painful, photophobic and there is profuse lacrimation. It is usually necessary to instil a drop of local anaesthetic (benoxinate or amethocaine) to examine the eye properly.

The foreign body is readily seen, with the aid of a pen torch, as a dark opacity in the superficial cornea. If it has been present for more than a few hours it is likely to be surrounded by a 'rust ring', which is caused by staining of the adjacent corneal stroma.

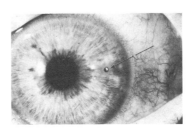
Corneal foreign body.

Causes

Most persistent corneal foreign bodies strike the eye at fairly high speed. Common causes are hammering, drilling and grinding.

Management

Following the instillation of a drop of local anaesthetic a superficial corneal foreign body can be removed, under suitable magnification, with a sterile, hypodermic needle. If a 'rust ring' is present this is left for 24–48 hours after which time it will easily lift away. Following removal of the foreign body or 'rust ring', antibiotic ointment and a cycloplegic drop (for example cyclopentolate 1%) are instilled and the eye covered with a pad.

Subtarsal foreign body

Clinical features

Small foreign bodies which blow into the eye are usually washed away by the tears. Occasionally one will become embedded in the subtarsal conjunctiva of the upper eyelid causing pain and fine, vertically linear, corneal abrasions on blinking.

Management

The upper eyelid is everted and the foreign body removed with a cotton wool bud or the edge of a paper tissue. Antibiotic ointment is instilled but a pad is not required. The foreign body sensation may persist for a short time after its removal.

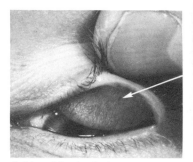

Subtarsal foreign body.

Corneal abrasion

Clinical features

The pain and watering of a corneal abrasion are rapidly relieved by a drop of local anaesthetic. With the aid of a pen torch the area of epithelial loss is visible as a disturbance of the corneal reflex but may be more easily seen with the aid of fluorescein.

Causes

Twigs, babies' fingernails and the edge of a piece of paper are common causes of corneal abrasions.

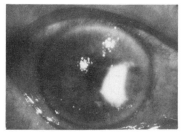

Corneal abrasion stained with fluorescein.

Management

Antibiotic ointment and a longer acting cycloplegic drop, such as homatropine 2%, are instilled and the eye is covered with a pad and bandage. The defect is rapidly covered by sliding of the adjacent epithelium and most abrasions are healed within 48 hours.

Occasionally healing of an abrasion is imperfect leading to a *recurrent corneal erosion*. The symptoms and management are the same as for the original lesion.

A blow to the eye, for example from a fist or ball, may cause a variety of ocular injuries represented in the composite diagram.

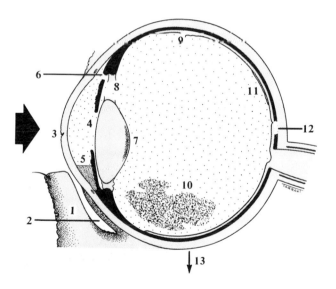

1. 'Black' eye
This is a haematoma within the soft tissues of the lids which may spread down over the cheek. The swelling and discoloration resolve within 2 weeks.

2. Subconjunctival haemorrhage
This appears as a bright red patch through the transparent conjunctiva. It is limited anteriorly by the attachment of the conjunctiva at the corneal limbus.

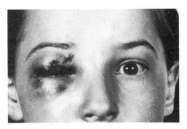

Black eye.

3. Corneal abrasion

A blow to the eye may remove corneal epithelium but often the quick reflex closure of the lids prevents this. In exceptionally severe trauma the cornea may rupture at the limbus.

4. Traumatic mydriasis

Paralysis of the pupil is commonly found after severe trauma and may be permanent. Rupture of the iris sphincter muscle may be visible as irregularity of the pupil margin.

5. Hyphaema

This is one of the commonest consequences of trauma to the eye. Damage to the iris blood vessels causes haemorrhage into the anterior chamber. Initially the blood is dispersed through the aqueous, reducing vision and impeding ophthalmoscopic examination of the fundus. Within a short period of time the blood, which does not readily clot in aqueous, settles in the lower part of the anterior chamber with the formation of a fluid level.

Most hyphaemas disperse within a few days but if the anterior chamber is filled with blood (a so-called 'eight-ball' hyphaema on account of the black appearance of the cornea) glaucoma and blood staining of the cornea may occur. Surgical removal of the blood is then necessary.

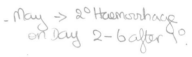

Traumatic mydriasis, rupture of iris sphincter (A), and hyphaema (B).

6. Iridodialysis

Tearing of the root of the iris from the ciliary body causes distortion of the pupil but vision may be little impaired once the accompanying hyphaema has dispersed.

Occasionally the ciliary body itself may be separated from the sclera giving rise to 'angle recession'. This damage to the drainage angle of the eye may give rise to *glaucoma*, sometimes developing several years after the injury.

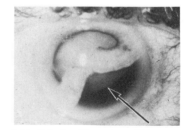

Iridodialysis with tearing of iris sphincter. Note edge of dislocated cataractous lens (arrowed).

7. Concussion cataract

This may progress to significant opacification and require removal of the lens.

8. Lens subluxation

The zonule supporting the lens may rupture causing subluxation or occasionally complete dislocation. The former produces distorted and reduced vision, the latter the state of aphakia. The iris is tremulous (iridodonesis) due to loss of the normal support given by the lens.

9. Retinal tear

This is particularly likely to occur in predisposed eyes with areas of retinal weakness (especially high myopes). Treatment is required to prevent the development of a retinal detachment.

10. Vitreous haemorrhage

There is frequently an associated retinal tear and careful examination of the fundus is essential once an adequate view can be obtained through the haemorrhage.

11. Commotio retinae

Striking the globe can cause a 'contra-coup' injury resulting in oedema and haemorrhage of the retina at the point opposite the site of impact. This may resolve without complication but more severe injuries result in visual loss with scarring and pigmentary disturbance.

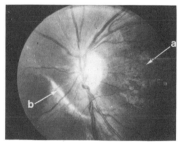

12. Choroidal rupture

Severe compression of the eye may rupture the choroid. Once the haemorrhage has resolved white crescentic scars are visible, usually close to the optic nerve. If the overlying retina is damaged, especially in the macular region, visual loss is severe.

Commotio retinae (*a*) and choroidal rupture (*b*).

13. Blow-out fracture

Posterior displacement of the globe may so elevate the orbital pressure that the bony orbit breaks at its weakest point. This is usually the orbital floor and herniation of soft tissues into the maxillary sinus occurs.

Clinical features include: (1) enophthalmos (a sunken eye) which may be difficult to diagnose while the lids are swollen, (2) restriction of eye movement,

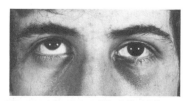

Blow-out fracture of the left orbit—attempted upgaze.

especially on upward gaze, giving rise to diplopia, and (3) loss of sensation over the regions supplied by the infra-orbital nerve.

Sinus x-rays show clouding of the affected sinus but tomography is usually required to demonstrate the fracture and herniation of orbital tissue.

Management is governed by the presence of any associated injuries. Surgical intervention to repair the fracture and replace the orbital contents depends on the severity of the enophthalmos and the likelihood of spontaneous resolution of diplopia.

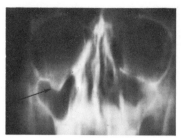

Tomogram of right blow-out fracture.

Penetrating injuries

23

Penetrating injuries of the eye are easily overlooked when:

1. An adequate history of the injury is not taken.
2. A patient presents with trauma to other parts of the head and face.

Failure to make the diagnosis may lead to loss of the eye and is a frequent cause of litigation.

Corneoscleral lacerations

Clinical features
Laceration of the cornea frequently results in prolapse of the iris with distortion of the pupil. A hyphaema is often present and vision is reduced. If the sclera is involved there may be severe intraocular haemorrhage from damage to the ciliary body. Perforation of the lens capsule results in cataract formation.

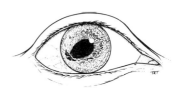

Corneal laceration with iris prolapse and distorted pupil.

Causes
Most corneoscleral lacerations are caused by glass. Shattered spectacles and broken windows or windscreens are common causes.

Management
In any penetrating injury of the globe it is a wise precaution to take an x-ray to exclude a retained foreign body. Surgical repair of the wound is undertaken to restore the integrity of the eye as far as possible. The risk of intraocular infection is often low but prophylactic antibiotics are routinely given.

111

Intraocular foreign body (IOFB)

Clinical features

The patient is usually aware of something having struck the eye but in the early stages there may be no significant visual loss. The history, however, will usually indicate whether a foreign body is likely to have entered the eye.

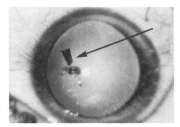

IOFB embedded in lens causing cataract.

Cause

This is usually a small piece of metal that has struck the eye at high velocity. A common cause is a hammer and chisel injury—a small flake may fly off either the head of the hammer or the head of the steel chisel as the former strikes the latter. *The penetrating wound and intraocular foreign body may be easily missed and an x-ray of the orbit is essential if such an injury is described.*

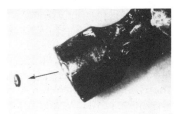

IOFB from hammer head.

Management

The risk of infection is relatively low unless the eye is penetrated by vegetable material. Systemic antibiotic therapy may be required in addition to topical treatment and the possiblity of fungal infection should be borne in mind.

Retained metallic foreign bodies, especially those containing iron and copper, give rise to serious chemical reaction within the eye. *Siderosis* from iron causes staining of the iris, cataract and retinal atrophy leading to blindness over a period of months while *chalcosis* from copper causes an acute inflammatory reaction within the eye (endophthalmitis) leading to rapid loss of vision.

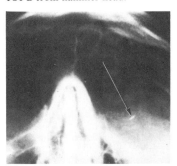

X-ray of IOFB.

Ferrous intraocular foreign bodies are removed with the aid of a powerful electromagnet. Non-magnetic foreign bodies are removed mechanically with the aid of fine forceps. X-ray localization of a radio-opaque foreign body is frequently necessary because of the presence of cataract or vitreous haemorrhage.

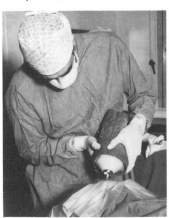

Electromagnetic removal of IOFB.

Sympathetic ophthalmitis

A penetrating injury of one eye may result in a sympathizing inflammatory reaction in the fellow, non-injured eye at any time from 2 weeks to many years later. This was one of the first autoimmune diseases to be recognized.

A prerequisite of sympathetic ophthalmitis is the involvement of the uveal tract, particularly the ciliary body, in the initiating injury. It is thought that release of uveal pigment into the bloodstream causes antibodies to be produced which result in a severe uveitis in both the injured and non-injured eye. If the injured eye is removed within 2 weeks of the injury the risk of this condition developing are greatly reduced. Such action is usually undertaken when there is no chance of saving useful vision and the injured eye remains inflamed. Systemic steroids greatly modify the course of this disease which otherwise may end in total blindness.

24

Chemical, thermal and radiation injuries

Chemical injuries

Clinical features

The extent of the ocular damage depends on the concentration of the chemical and the speed with which the eye is irrigated. Usually there is intense blepharospasm and the lids can only be separated with difficulty. Conjunctival damage may lead to the formation of adhesions and corneal damage may result in opacification. Alkalis penetrate the cornea more easily than acids and can cause severe intraocular inflammation with cataract formation.

- adhesions = Symblephreon.

alkali → Saponification →Penet

Acid → ppt of protein →Barrier

Causes

The majority of injuries are industrial and can be prevented by the wearing of protective goggles. Concentrated sulphuric acid from exploding car batteries and ammonia used in criminal assault are not uncommon causes of severe bilateral ocular injury.

Management

Immediate and copious irrigation with water is essential. This should be repeated on arrival of the patient in the Casualty Department. Topical antibiotics are essential to prevent the development of secondary infection and steroids may be required to suppress intraocular inflammation. Vitamin C, both in drop and tablet form, has a role in the limitation of corneal damage. Conjunctival grafting from the fellow eye may aid re-epithelization in severely injured eyes; corneal grafting has a low success rate.

1. Antibiotics
2 Steroids
3. Anticholinergics
4 Vit C - High conc -Oral +
Drops

114

Thermal injuries

Clinical features

Minor burns of the conjunctiva and cornea cause coagulation of the epithelium with the appearance of white marks. More serious burns usually involve the eyelids as well and there may be serious ocular sequelae as a result of lid scarring.

Causes

1. MINOR BURNS

Hot fat and lighted cigarettes are common causes.

2. SEVERE

These are usually the result of fires or explosions.

Management

1. MINOR

There is rapid re-epithelization of the burnt area. Antibiotic ointment and a cycloplegic drop are instilled and the eye covered with a pad.

2. SEVERE

Treatment is initially directed towards protection of the cornea from exposure and consequent ulceration and infection. Plastic surgery to the eyelids may be required.

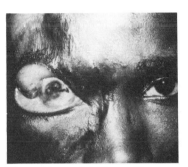

Thermal burn of right eye with ectropion and corneal scarring.

Radiation injuries

Ionizing radiation

Clinical features

All the tissues of the eye may be involved. The skin of the lids becomes atrophic and the eyelashes are lost. Scarring of the conjunctiva leads to a dry eye with secondary corneal damage and the lens becomes cataractous. Retinal and optic atrophy are the consequence of ischaemic changes in the posterior segment of the eye.

Causes

Radiotherapy is by far the commonest cause.

Management

This is directed towards treatment of the dry eye and, if necessary, removal of the cataract.

Ultraviolet light

Clinical features

Exposure to high levels of ultraviolet light results in a painful punctate keratitis. There is profuse lacrimation and mild conjunctival hyperaemia.

Causes

1. Solar. Reflected light from snow, sea or sand
2. Sunlamps
3. Welding flashes

Management

Spontaneous resolution occurs within 36 hours. Topical anaesthetics provide instantaneous relief from the pain, and may be necessary for adequate examination of the eye, but their repeated use may result in serious corneal damage. Homatropine 2% drops, to relieve ciliary spasm, and padding of the eyes are usually sufficient.

Solar burns

Intense light, within the visible spectrum, focused on the retina will produce a burn. This is the principle of retinal photocoagulation. Visual loss may be the result of a macula burnt by looking at the sun ('eclipse burn') without adequate protection from dark filters.

Part 2

The eye in systemic disease

Background Retinopathy

1. Dil, bleeding + tortuosity of R. Veins
2. Microaneurysms   - often temporal to Macula.
3. Hard exudates   - often be in O's   due to lipid in Macrophages.
4. Cotton Wool Spots
5. Retinal oedema   - due to Axoplasm
6. Intra Retinal Microvascular ab⊕.
7. Haemorrhage - Dot / Blot

Maculopathy.
Macular Oedema   Mj. cause of Loss of Vision in D.M. pts.

1. Oedema of Retina at the Macula   - Vision Compromised ->6/60
2. Leakage from retinal Capillaries at the Macula.   -> Vessels obliterated.
3. Cystoid Δ in Retina.
4. Exudates
5. Exudative plaque.

Proliferative Retinopathy

1. new vessels at the optic disc
2. flat retinal new vessels
3. forward retinal new vessels
4. Retinitis Proliferans   - with fibrous tissue

Factors for severe Visual Loss in D. Retinopathy

1. Vitreous or preretinal Haemorrhage
2. New vessels
3. Optic Disc new vessels.
4. Severity of new vessels.

No. of Factors	Rate
1	6.7%
2	8.5%
3	26.7%
4	36.9%

Cumulative ↑ Risk.

Advanced Diabetic eye Disease.

1. Proliferative Diabetic Retinopathy
2. Vitreous Haemorrhage.
3. Intra vitreal fibrous tissue - Vitreous Traction bands.
4. Traction retinal detachment.
5. Rhegmatogenous Retinal detachment
6. Rubeosis Iridis.
7. Rubeosis Glaucoma.

Diabetes mellitus

As the life expectancy of diabetics has increased with improved treatment so has the incidence of major complications including loss of vision. In the developed world diabetic retinopathy is now the leading cause of blindness in adults under the age 65.

Diabetes can affect almost all the structures of the eye but most commonly involved are the retina and lens.

Diabetic retinopathy

Pathogenesis

Diabetic retinopathy is a microvascular disease. Weakening of capillaries results in microaneurysm formation, retinal haemorrhage and transudation of fluid and lipid while progressive capillary obliteration gives rise to areas of retinal ischaemia. In turn this leads to the formation of new vessels on the surface of the retina and iris. It is postulated that ischaemic retina forms a vasoproliferative substance though this has not been identified.

Clinical features

1. BACKGROUND DIABETIC RETINOPATHY
Microaneurysms are the earliest sign of diabetic retinopathy, later accompanied by discrete intraretinal ('dot and blot') haemorrhages and scattered hard exudates. These changes are most marked in the posterior retina but may be compatible with normal vision. This type of retinopathy is found mainly in elderly diabetics who have had the disease for several years.

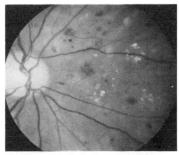

Background diabetic retinopathy.

2. DIABETIC MACULOPATHY

Gradual loss of vision in a patient with non-proliferative diabetic retinopathy is usually due to macular disease. This may be caused by:

a. Capillary leakage giving rise to chronic macular oedema.
b. Lipid deposition in the macular area.
c. Extensive obliteration of the macular capillaries.

3. PROLIFERATIVE RETINOPATHY

This type of retinopathy is seen most frequently in young patients on insulin therapy who have had the disease for at least ten years. New vessels develop from the venous side of the circulation on the optic disc and the surface of the retina adjacent the temporal vessels. These vessels bleed, causing either preretinal or vitreous haemorrhage which may obscure the vision for months or even years. Later, glial tissue may form around these vessels and contracture gives rise to a traction retinal detachment.

Diabetic retinopathy may also lead to the development of neovascular ('thrombotic') glaucoma. New blood vessels, accompanied by a sheet of fibrous tissue, develop on the surface of the iris and obstruct the drainage angle.

Management

No specific treatment is required for background diabetic retinopathy if vision is unaffected.

If visual acuity falls a fluorescein angiogram may help determine the type of maculopathy present. Laser photocoagulation may reduce macular oedema and preserve vision but is of no benefit where there is extensive capillary closure. Exudates involving the macula may be successfully treated, particularly when they occur as part of a ring surrounding an area of focal retinal ischaemia. Laser treatment is applied to the centre of the ring.

The mainstay of treatment of proliferative retinopathy is photocoagulation of the retina either by argon laser or xenon arc light. Treatment is directed not at the new vessels themselves but is spread over a wide area of the retina (pan-retinal photocoagulation). It is believed that extensive destruction of ischaemic retina prevents the formation of the vasoproliferative factor. Clinically, regression of the new vessels is seen. Treatment of the peripheral retina in this manner leads

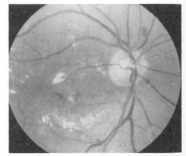
Diabetic maculopathy.

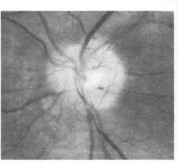
a, New vessels arising from optic disc.

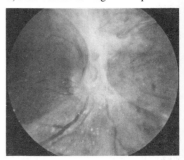
b, Advanced proliferative retinopathy.

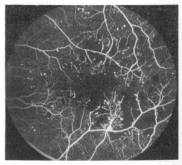
Fluorescein angiogram of diabetic maculopathy showing microaneurysms and capillary closure.

to varying degrees of visual field loss and 'night blindness' but it is often possible to preserve good central vision and useful visual field if treatment is given at a time when new vessel formation is reversible.

With the development of sophisticated operating microscopes and instruments which can be passed into the vitreous cavity, methods are now available for the removal of persistent vitreous haemorrhage and treatment of traction detachments.

Neovascular glaucoma may be prevented by pan-retinal photocoagulation but the established disease is very difficult to control. Eyes that are blind from neovascular glaucoma are frequently painful. Symptomatic relief may be obtained with atropine and steroid drops but failing this nerve block with retro-ocular alcohol injection or even enucleation (removal of the eye) may be necessary.

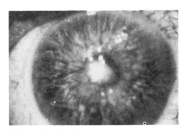
Thrombotic glaucoma—new vessels on surface of iris seen through corneal oedema.

Cataract

Cataracts of the senile type occur more frequently in diabetics. Surgical removal is accompanied by an increased rate of complications and the visual result is frequently compromised by the presence of maculopathy.

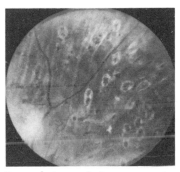
Laser photocoagulation scars.

Occasionally, in young insulin-dependent diabetics, a cataract with white flecks may develop rapidly. This 'true' diabetic cataract is occasionally reversible in the very early stages.

Poorly controlled diabetics may experience a fluctuation of their vision, which parallels the level of blood sugar.

Cranial nerve palsies

Elderly diabetics may develop palsies affecting the oculomotor nerves. The onset is acute and painful and full recovery can take several months. A third nerve palsy is the most common; pupillary dilatation is usually *absent*. also CN VI

assoc with unilateral headache

Thyroid disease

Thyrotoxicosis (Graves' disease) is a common condition, which affects women more frequently than men. In classical Graves' disease the eyes are prominent with a degree of lid retraction and lid lag. These features are mild and are of no great consequence and resolve when the condition is treated.

In a minority of cases serious ophthalmic complications develop (dysthyroid eye disease or ophthalmic Graves' disease). This can occur in any thyroid state but is most commonly seen after the treatment of thyrotoxicosis. An autoimmune reaction occurs in the orbit causing oedema and lymphocytic infiltration of both the orbital fat and muscles and the clinical features of the disease stem from this.

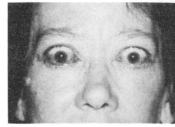

Ophthalmic Graves' disease.

Proptosis = forward protrusion of the eye + lid

Dysthyroid eye disease is the *commonest cause of both unilateral and bilateral proptosis*. The proptosis can vary from mild to extreme. The eyelids are thickened and oedematous, the conjunctiva is swollen (chemotic) and deep vertical furrows are seen in the forehead at the base of the nose. Lid cover of the cornea may be inadequate causing exposure and ulceration; lateral tarsorrhaphy may be required. In severe cases vision may be threatened by corneal exposure or optic nerve compression; urgent treatment to relieve the raised orbital pressure is required and this may be achieved by the use of systemic steroids, by surgical decompression of the orbit or occasionally by radiotherapy.

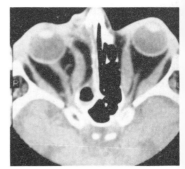

CT scan of dysthyroid eye disease with thickened extraocular muscles and proptosis.

Diplopia

The extraocular muscles are swollen to several times their normal dimensions. This can be clearly demonstrated on a CT scan and is helpful in distinguishing this condition from other causes of proptosis. Limitation of ocular movement is a consequence of secondary fibrotic changes within the muscles and this affects particularly the inferior rectus muscle. This gives rise to vertical diplopia which is most marked on upward gaze. Muscle surgery to realign the eyes is undertaken when the condition is stable.

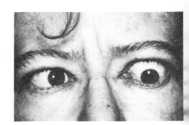

Proptosis and limitation of elevation of the left eye.

Management

Treatment of dysthyroid eye disease is aimed at preventing serious ocular complications and relieving symptoms, as outlined above. The pathogenesis of the condition is poorly understood and treatment to alter thyroid function, when abnormal, has no significant effect on the course of the eye disease.

Dysthyroid eye disease is a self-limiting condition but resolution of the proptosis and muscle changes is at best only partial. However, there is seldom reactivation of the disease.

Pituitary tumours

Pituitary tumours present either as an endocrine deficiency state or as a cause of visual loss. They seldom cause raised intracranial pressure.

Pituitary adenomas

Pituitary adenomas are not rare. Although the great majority are histologically benign they slowly enlarge and expand the sella. The weakest part of this structure is the roof so that expansion is mainly upwards affecting the optic chiasm. The central fibres (from the nasal half of each retina) are first involved producing the hallmark of chiasmal compression which is *bitemporal hemianopia*. At this stage the diagnosis is often missed as many patients do not appreciate the nature of the visual loss and visual acuity is normal.

Although the lateral walls of the cavernous sinus carry all the oculomotor nerves it is unusual for pituitary adenomas to cause double vision. However, in the rare event of haemorrhage into the gland the expansion is acute and oculomotor palsies may then arise. These tumours seldom cause raised intracranial pressure as there is space for expansion into the basal cisterns. The effect on the optic chiasm is to produce optic atrophy.

Chromophobe adenomas are the most common type and 80% develop ophthalmic features. Systemically there are signs of hypopituitarism and impotence or amenorrhoea may be the presenting complaint.

Acidophil adenomas cause acromegaly (or gigantism in children) and 25% cause ophthalmic signs. *Basophil* adenomas, which are rare and cause hypersecretion of the adrenal cortex, and prolactinomas, which are relatively common, only occasionally affect vision.

Craniopharyngiomas

These tumours arise from epithelial remnants in the pituitary stalk. They occur in both children and adults.

Endocrine deficiency states (dwarfism, hypogenitalism) are seen and diabetes insipidus may occur. In children the tumour may invade the third ventricle causing internal hydrocephalus with papilloedema.

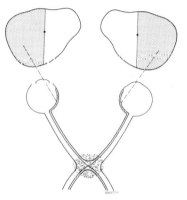

Bitemporal hemianopia.

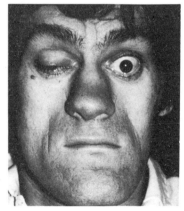

Acromegaly with right third nerve palsy due to pituitary apoplexy.

Management

The main aim of treatment is the preservation of vision by relief of chiasmal compression. A plain lateral skull x-ray, showing ballooning of the sella and erosion of the clinoid processes confirms the presence of an intrasellar lesion but CT scanning is valuable in determining the degree of suprasellar expansion. Surgical removal is usually followed by radiotherapy. Craniopharyngiomas are more difficult to remove owing to their close association with the hypothalamus and floor of the third ventricle.

Correction of any endocrine abnormality, caused by tumour or removal of the pituitary gland, is also required.

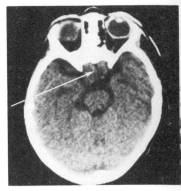

CT scan of pituitary tumour.

Vascular disease

Many diseases affecting the eye have a vascular cause. Pathological changes occurring within the retinal vascular tree can be directly observed allowing not only diagnosis of the local condition but also an assessment of the state of the vascular system as a whole.

The two conditions commonly underlying vascular disease of the eye are *hypertension* and *atheroma*. The former causes distinctive retinal vascular changes but the latter affects arteries of a larger calibre than the retinal arterioles. Ocular disease caused by atheroma is usually secondary to involvement of the carotid vessels.

Hypertension

The type of retinal vascular change occurring in hypertension depends on a number of factors including the duration of the disease, the age of the patient and the level of the blood pressure. The changes occurring in an elderly patient with essential hypertension are quite different from those in a young patient with accelerated hypertension.

Essential hypertension

This is associated with thickening of the arteriolar wall followed by hyaline degeneration and later narrowing of the lumen. Opthalmoscopically the normally transparent arteriole (only the column of red blood cells is visible) becomes progressively opaque with a heightened reflex from its surface ('*silver wiring*') and constriction of veins at the arteriovenous crossings (*AV nipping*). It should be noted that these

+ Angulation — esp. young

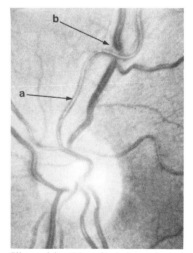

Silver wiring (*a*) and arteriovenous nipping (*b*).

arteriosclerotic changes may also be seen in normotensive elderly patients. Retinal haemorrhages may occur but if profuse these usually indicate an associated retinal vascular accident.

Accelerated (malignant) hypertension

The fundus picture tends to be more florid in younger patients in whom there is no 'protective' pre-existing sclerosis of the retinal arterioles. Narrowing and irregularity of the arterioles is accompanied by closure in the pre-capillary region causing small retinal infarcts (soft 'exudates' or *cotton-wool spots*). Superficial retinal haemorrhages are seen radiating away from the optic disc and hard exudates may surround the macula forming a partial or complete 'star'. *Papilloedema* is caused by vascular changes within the optic nerve head leading to swelling of the nerve fibres and leakage of fluid from the vessels. Retinal oedema at the posterior pole of the eye usually accompanies the papilloedema and if the macula is involved vision may be impaired.

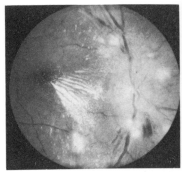

Malignant hypertension with partial macular star and retinal infarcts.

Ocular complications of hypertension include central and branch retinal vein occlusion, central and branch retinal artery occlusion, ischaemic optic neuropathy and vitreous haemorrhage.

Management

Treatment of hypertension results in clearing of the exudative changes if adequate control is maintained. Haemorrhages tend to absorb rapidly and cotton-wool spots usually resolve within a few weeks. Hard exudates take many months, and sometimes longer than a year, to disappear. Papilloedema may decrease rapidly but a grossly swollen disc may never return to normal and may eventually show signs of atrophy. As might be expected arteriolar changes are little influenced by controlling the blood pressure.

Atheroma

Atheroma may cause ophthalmic disease in one of two ways—either through the formation of emboli or by interfering with ocular and cerebral perfusion.

Embolization

Emboli originating from atheromatous plaques, usually at the origin of the internal carotid artery, may cause transient or permanent loss of vision.

Transient loss of vision (*amaurosis fugax*) is caused either by cholesterol or platelet emboli. The former are seen as small, refractile bodies often lodged at the bifurcation of a retinal arteriole. Platelet emboli are small, whitish bodies which pass rapidly through the retinal circulation causing repeated, very brief attacks of amaurosis fugax. Detached thrombus, which arises more commonly from the heart, produces a larger embolus which impacts either in the central retinal artery itself or at the first or second bifurcation. Permanent loss of vision is more common with this type of embolus.

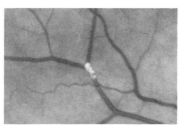

Cholesterol embolus.

Carotid occlusive disease

Carotid artery stenosis may also cause transient loss of vision through retinal ischaemia. If both carotid arteries are severely stenosed a fall in cardiac output will result in bilateral visual loss or 'blackout'. Unilateral stenosis may result in a clinical picture of amaurosis fugax almost indistinguishable from that caused by emboli.

Vertebrobasilar ischaemia

Ischaemia of the occipital cortex may result in transient visual phenomena , including visual field loss and other migraine-like symptoms. Occlusion of one posterior cerebral artery results in unilateral infarction of the occipital cortex and a homonymous hemianopia. Macular vision may or may not be spared. Bilateral infarction of the occipital cortex causes blindness which is often denied (Anton's syndrome).

Patients with vertebrobasilar disease may also present with transient or permanent double vision due to involvement of the ocular motor nerve nuclei and their connections in the brainstem. Other neurological features include facial paraesthesiae, vertigo, dysarthria and ataxia.

Management

Transient loss of vision always requires careful investigation as a treatable cause may be found. Carotid artery stenosis can be surgically corrected by endarterectomy with significant reduction in the risk of stroke. If endarterectomy is contraindicated anticoagulation may be employed.

Neurological disease 27

Neurological disease frequently produces ocular signs of diagnostic importance. Papilloedema, optic atrophy and visual field loss are discussed below; abnormalities of eye movement and pupil reactions are considered in earlier chapters.

Papilloedema

Papilloedema literally means swelling of the optic disc but the term is generally restricted to swelling caused by stasis rather than inflammation.

Swelling of the optic disc due to *raised intracranial pressure* is almost invariably bilateral. The optic nerves are covered with meninges and raised intracranial pressure is transmitted to the optic nerve head resulting in interruption of normal axoplasmic flow and the appearance of a choked disc.

The degree of disc swelling may vary considerably but consistent features are blurring of the disc margin and engorgement of the retinal veins. The disc itself is usually hyperaemic and there are commonly flame-shaped haemorrhages and cotton-wool spots on or immediately adjacent to the disc.

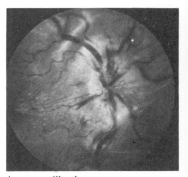

Acute papilloedema.

Acute papilloedema is compatible with normal vision though enlargement of the blind spot can be demonstrated and transient obscuration of vision occasionally occurs. Progressive optic atrophy and visual failure may occur if the condition becomes chronic.

Causes

1. Intracranial space-occupying lesions, including tumours, particularly of the posterior fossa, haematoma and cerebral abscess.

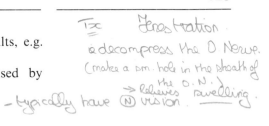

Handwritten note: Tx   Fenestration
& decompress the O Nerve.
(make a sm. hole in the sheath of
the O. N.)
→ Relieves swelling.
- typically have (N) vision.

2. Any lesion causing hydrocephalus in adults, e.g. meningitis and subarachnoid haemorrhage.
3. Venous obstruction which may be caused by thrombosis in the venous sinuses.
4. Benign intracranial hypertension.

Differential diagnosis

1. *Accelerated (malignant) hypertension.* Papilloedema is usually bilateral but accompanied by other features of hypertensive retinopathy. There is usually some degree of visual failure.

2. Other causes of papilloedema (usually *unilateral*), include central retinal vein occlusion, ischaemic optic neuropathy and optic neuritis. These are all accompanied by *sudden loss of vision.*

3. *Pseudopapilloedema.* Conditions which mimic papilloedema include the small disc with blurred margins found in *hypermetropia* and hyaline deposits (giant *drusen*) which form in the disc head. Fluorescein angiography is helpful in the differential diagnosis; leakage of fluorescein from dilated superficial capillaries occurs in papilloedema but not in pseudopapilloedema.

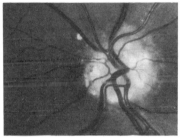

Pseudopapilloedema due to giant drusen.

Optic atrophy

Optic atrophy is caused by damage to the nerve fibres at any point between and including the ganglion cells of the retina and the lateral geniculate body. It is usually associated with loss of either central or peripheral vision but the correlation between visual loss and the degree of pallor may be poor.

The pallor of advanced optic atrophy is unmistakable but difficulty may be experienced in differentiating minor degrees of atrophy from variants of the normal disc. The central pallor of a large physiological cup (an area devoid of neural tissue through which the cribriform plate can be seen) and scleral exposure adjacent to the optic disc (often seen in the myopic eye) may confuse the inexperienced.

Atrophy is accompanied by attenuation of the retinal vessels and changes in visual acuity, colour vision, visual field and pupil reactions. If these are all normal it is unlikely that pallor of the optic disc is pathological though an abnormality of the visually

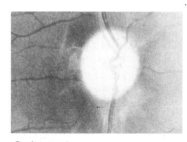

Optic atrophy.

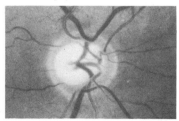

Central pallor of disc due to large physiological cup.

evoked response (VER) may be the only confirmation of a previous episode of optic nerve demyelination.

Once optic atrophy is established the appearance does not return to normal even if the cause is relieved; visual function, however, may recover.

The causes of optic atrophy include:

1. Retinal

a. Central retinal artery occlusion.
b. Retinal abiotrophies (e.g. retinitis pigmentosa).
c. Toxic, e.g. from quinine or methyl alcohol poisoning.

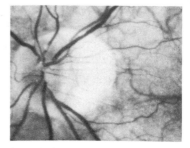

Myopic disc with scleral crescent.

2. Optic nerve

a. Ischaemic optic neuropathy.
b. Optic and retrobulbar neuritis.
c. Chronic glaucoma. This is the commonest cause of optic atrophy but differs from others in one important respect. In glaucomatous atrophy there is progressive loss of neural and supporting glial tissue leading to excavation of the nerve head. This rarely happens in optic atrophy from other causes.
d. Consecutive to papilloedema. (chronic)
e. Toxic, e.g. methyl alcohol, ethyl alcohol, tobacco and ethambutol.
f. Deficiency diseases, e.g. pernicious anaemia.
g. Tumour. Optic nerve glioma or meningioma.
h. Trauma.
i. Hereditary optic atrophy.

3. Chiasm

Any cause of chiasmal compression (*see below*).

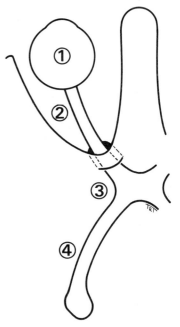

Sites of lesions causing optic atrophy.

4. Optic tract

An uncommon site for the production of optic atrophy. The tract is most commonly involved, along with the chiasm, in compression due to a pituitary adenoma.

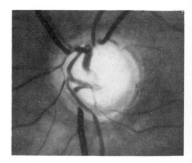

Glaucomatous atrophy.

Visual field loss

The widespread course of the visual pathway through the brain results in visual loss from a great diversity of neurological disease. The nature of the visual loss frequently indicates the site of the lesion but less often the actual cause.

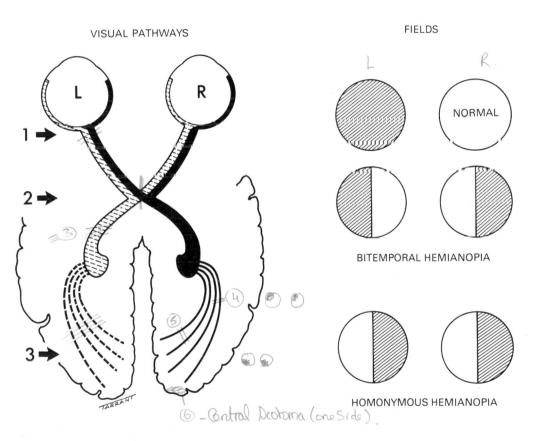

VISUAL PATHWAYS

FIELDS

NORMAL

BITEMPORAL HEMIANOPIA

HOMONYMOUS HEMIANOPIA

⑥ – Central Scotoma (one side).

1. The eye and optic nerve

Visual loss in one eye only is caused by disease anterior to the optic chiasm. The main causes have been considered in those chapters dealing with sudden and gradual loss of vision.

Central loss of vision suggests macular or optic nerve disease. Peripheral field loss in one eye may be due to retinal disease, e.g. detachment or vascular occlusion, or disease of the optic nerve head such as chronic glaucoma or ischaemic optic neuropathy.

④ +⑤ – Because the optic Radiation fans out partial / Quadrantic defects are more common!

2. Optic chiasm

Lesions affecting the chiasm cause bitemporal hemianopia though this is frequently asymmetrical. Visual acuity may be affected early or late in the course of the compression but eventually the entire chiasm is involved resulting in complete blindness.

3. Optic tract and radiation

Lesions posterior to the chiasm cause homonymous field loss on the opposite side.

Lesions of the optic tracts are uncommon and are usually caused by posterior extension of pituitary adenomas.

Hence /> optic Atrophy

Lesions of the optic radiations are common, particularly those caused by tumours and vascular accidents. The field loss is frequently mistaken by the patient for loss of vision in one eye rather than loss of half the field in both eyes. Visual acuity is usually normal due to sparing of the macular area.

- Stroke !

The field loss in each eye may be identical (congruous) suggesting a posterior lesion near the occipital cortex. If the field loss is markedly different in the two eyes (incongruous) the lesion is more anteriorly placed.

X Chiasmal compression

-> See Down Nystagmus

The nerve fibres within the chiasm can be affected by a variety of conditions arising from neighbouring structures. Compression of the chiasm is not uncommon and is frequently missed in the early stages. The clinical features are pathognomonic and consist of bitemporal hemianopia, loss of visual acuity and optic atrophy.

Progressive bitemporal hemianopia

It is only at the chiasm that lesions can produce this pattern of field loss owing to the decussation of the nasal fibres of each optic nerve.

Loss of visual acuity and optic atrophy

As the visual field loss advances the acuity becomes steadily worse and poor colour vision may be noticed by the patient. The optic discs become progressively paler but papilloedema does not occur as there is space for the lesion to expand in the chiasmal cistern without raising the intracranial pressure.

Double vision is uncommon but may occur if the lesion causing chiasmal compression extends to involve the ocular motor nerves within the cavernous sinus.

Causes include:

1. Pituitary tumours.
2. Craniopharyngiomas.
3. Suprasellar meningiomas.

Less commonly:

4. Aneurysms.
5. Vascular accidents.
6. Trauma.

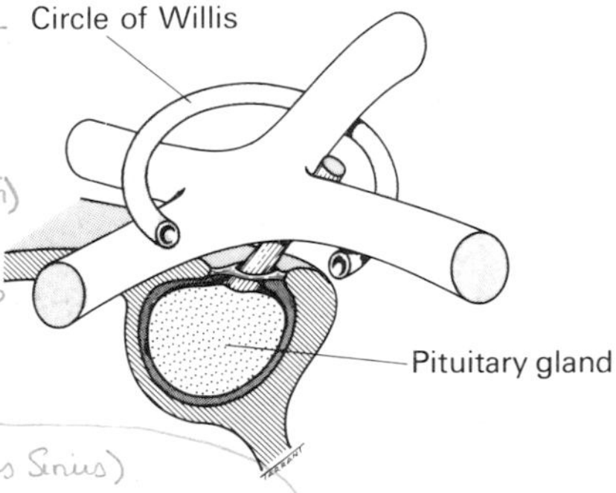

(handwritten annotations: V. Loss from Above ↓; (Chromophobe ± secrete Prolactin) (GH / ACTH). Visual loss from Below up; infra clinoid aneurysm (↑ size in Cavernous Sinus) → press on CN Ⅴ Chiasm → ↑ Pain in face!)

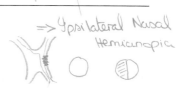

Circle of Willis

Pituitary gland

Optic chiasm and related structures.

(handwritten annotations: Meningiomas — sphenoidal Ridge, Olfactory groove, Tuberculum Sellae)

Ocular motor nerve palsies

The third, fourth and sixth cranial nerves may be affected by a variety of neurological diseases at any point from the brainstem to the orbit.

(handwritten annotations: ⇒ Ypsilateral Nasal Hemianopia; LR₆ (DO₄). others CN Ⅲ — MR. SR. IR. IO)

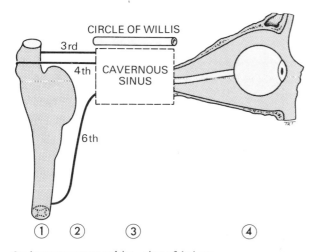

Ocular motor nerve palsies—sites of lesions.

1. Brainstem

Brainstem vascular accident, demyelinating lesion or tumour may cause an ocular muscle palsy. Coincidental involvement of other brainstem structures results in a variety of syndromes with ocular motor and long tract signs.

2. Lesions within the subarachnoid space

Raised intracranial pressure from any cause can produce a sixth nerve palsy which therefore has no localizing value in diagnosis.

The commonest intracranial cause of a third nerve palsy is aneurysm of the posterior communicating artery which lies just above the nerve before its entry into the cavernous sinus.

Fourth nerve palsies, frequently bilateral, occur as a result of closed head injury but are otherwise uncommon.

Other diseases affecting the intracranial portion of the ocular motor nerves include diabetes mellitus, herpes zoster and meningitis. Diabetes is a relatively common cause; the onset is usually painful and recovery the rule. If the third nerve is involved the pupil is usually 'spared'.

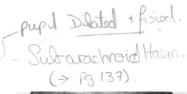

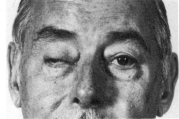

Right third nerve palsy.

3. Cavernous sinus

Pituitary tumours expand slowly and cranial nerve palsies are uncommon. However, sudden expansion with haemorrhage into the pituitary gland (pituitary apoplexy) can affect any or all three nerves.

Similarly, the development of an intracavernous carotid aneurysm causes a sudden, painful and total ophthalmoplegia.

4. Orbit

Nerve palsies result mainly from lesions around the superior orbital fissure and causes include trauma and meningiomas

Conditions such as orbital cellulitis, dysthyroid eye disease and orbital tumours tend to affect the muscles rather than the nerves.

Myasthenia gravis

This chronic, relatively uncommon disease affects the neuromuscular junction of skeletal muscles causing fatigue on effort.

Ocular features may be independent of generalized disease. The most common sign is unilateral or bilateral ptosis which tends to come on late in the day. Ophthalmoplegia may occur giving rise to variable diplopia; this may affect a single muscle or groups of muscles. The intrinsic muscles of the eye are rarely, if ever, affected.

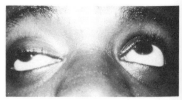

Ptosis and defective eye movement in myasthenia gravis.

Diagnosis

A marked and rapid improvement in signs follows intravenous injection of edrophonium chloride (Tensilon); demonstration of acetylcholine receptor antibodies confirms the diagnosis.

≡ Anticholinesterase

Management

Anticholinesterase drugs, such as neostigmine and pyridostigmine, are effective but the response may gradually decrease with the development of a fixed muscle palsy. Squint surgery may then be necessary.

About 10% of patients with myasthenia gravis have a thymoma. Thymectomy may be helpful, particularly in younger patients.

Use Neostigmine

-Later
= → Fixed Muscle palsy
→ Squint Surgery !

Thymectomy !

Horner's syndrome

This is caused by any interruption of the sympathetic pathway from the hypothalamus to the orbit. The clinical features include miosis of the pupil, slight ptosis (due to paralysis of the sympathetically innervated Müller's muscle) and loss of sweating over the forehead.

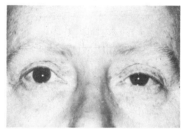

Horner's syndrome left ptosis.

Miosis, - slight
ptosis, - slight
↓ Sweating
heterochromia.
elevation of lower lid.
Hypotony
↑ amplitude of accommodation.

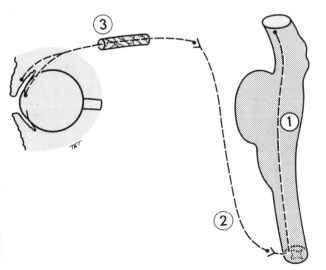

Horner's syndrome sites of lesions.

Causes

1. Within the central nervous system.

a. Vascular lesions, e.g. thrombosis of the posterior inferior cerebellar artery.
b. Demyelinating disease.
c. Space-occupying lesions.

2. Between thoracic outlet and superior cervical ganglion.

a. Pancoast tumour.   *Car of lung ass c̄ Horners synd.*
b. Cervical rib.
c. Thyroid enlargement.

3. Distal to superior cervical ganglion (post-ganglionic).

a. Injuries to the neck including surgical exploration and carotid arteriography.

Diagnosis

Cocaine drops (4%) dilate the normal pupil but not one affected by Horner's syndrome. Weak adrenaline drops do not affect the normal pupil but produce marked dilatation in Horner's syndrome when the lesion is postganglionic (above the superior cervical ganglion).

Facial palsy

Facial palsy is a common condition frequently occurring without an obvious cause (Bell's palsy). Within a short period of time the lower lid sags (lagophthalmos) and the upper lid may not descend sufficiently to cover the cornea (*see* Chapter 12). Other causes of facial palsy include brainstem vascular accidents, cerebellar pontine tumours and sarcoid.

Cerebrovascular accidents

Stroke

The major ophthalmic feature of stroke is involvement of the optic radiations giving rise to a homonymous hemianopia on the opposite side. Recovery can occur but it is not the rule. Patients may learn to compensate for the defect though reading usually remains difficult if the field defect is right sided. Homonymous hemianopia is a bar to driving.

If the pre-striate areas are involved dyslexia and gaze palsies may occur.

(Striae = Parts of 1° Cortex)

Subarachnoid haemorrhage

This condition presents with a devastating headache. The sudden leakage of blood into the cerebrospinal fluid causes an acute rise in intracranial pressure which may result in haemorrhage from the retinal vessels and frequently papilloedema. The haemorrhages lift the membrane which separates retina from vitreous and typically have a horizontal fluid level when the patient is upright (a 'subhyaloid' haemorrhage). Occasionally the haemorrhage breaks through into the vitreous.

Subarachnoid haemorrhage is most commonly caused by an aneurysm, especially of the posterior communicating artery which often produces an associated third nerve palsy.

↳ pupil dilated + fixed !

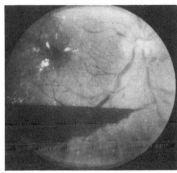

Subhyaloid haemorrhage (exudates at macula due to diabetes).

↳ deep to vitreous

Subhyaloid Haem. ②Vit.

Multiple sclerosis

The most common ocular manifestations of this common, progressive and untreatable disease are the result of demyelination of the optic nerve and brainstem.

Optic (retrobulbar) neuritis

By far the commonest cause of optic neuritis is demyelinating disease. It is often the presenting feature of multiple sclerosis but many patients who present with an isolated attack of optic neuritis do not develop further signs of demyelination.

The clinical features of optic and retrobulbar neuritis have been considered in the chapter on sudden loss of vision. It is worth noting that with repeated attacks optic atrophy develops and recovery of vision becomes less complete. Simultaneous bilateral attacks are uncommon but there is usually involvement of both eyes at some stage.

~ Central Scotoma

Episodes of demyelination posterior to the optic nerves will produce characteristic visual field defects.

Internuclear ophthalmoplegia

A demyelinating lesion of the medial longitudinal bundle causes internuclear ophthalmoplegia. The usual presentation is diplopia and on attempted lateral gaze the adducting eye fails to move beyond the midline. The abducting eye develops horizontal ('ataxic') nystagmus. In multiple sclerosis internuclear ophthalmoplegia is frequently bilateral. The medial recti, however, act normally in convergence. Recovery usually occurs though some degree of 'ataxic' nystagmus may persist.

Jerk nystagmus is a common finding in patients with multiple sclerosis and follows repeated episodes of brainstem demyelination.

MCQ. -pg 184.

─ a feature of Anti Convulsant Tox.
Disseminated Sclerosis
Wernicke's Encephalopathy.
Pontine Gliomas.

See Saw Nystagmus
ⁱ Chiasmal lesion

The phakomatoses

A group of uncommon congenital disorders affecting blood vessels and neural tissue. These hamartomas are histologically benign but can cause serious general and ophthalmic disease.

Neurofibromatosis (von Recklinghausen's disease)

Neurofibromas within the orbit may cause severe proptosis and visual failure. Multiple lesions in the upper lid (plexiform neuroma) produce a major cosmetic deformity. Optic nerve gliomas, usually presenting in childhood, may occur in association with neurofibromatosis though signs of the latter may be restricted to areas of cutaneous pigmentation (café-au-lait spots). These gliomas tend to be slow growing and relatively benign.

An acoustic neuroma is another manifestation of this disease which may affect the eye. As the tumour expands it causes deafness, facial weakness and anaesthesia in the distribution of the fifth nerve. During surgical removal the facial nerve is often sacrificed or damaged and the patient is left with an eye which cannot be closed and may have no sensation. This combination frequently results in corneal scarring and loss of vision.

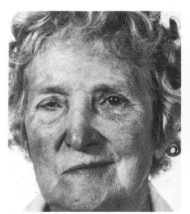

Acoustic neuroma with right facial palsy. A lateral tarsorrhaphy has been performed.

Sturge–Weber syndrome

The external manifestation of this disease is a haemangioma (port-wine stain) in the distribution of the trigeminal nerve. It is frequently associated with

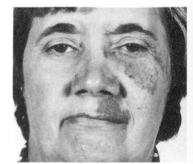

Port-wine stain in Sturge–Weber syndrome.

glaucoma on the affected side; orbital haemangiomas can cause proptosis. The meningeal vessels 'underneath' the skin or scalp lesion may be involved and result in fits, hemiplegia or even mental retardation. X-rays demonstrate calcification of the vessels which appear like tramlines.

Tuberous sclerosis (Bourneville's disease)

Large tumours develop in the central nervous system and cause mental retardation and death in early adult life. The 'tubers' are easily seen on a CT scan.

Retinal and optic nerve tumours have a characteristic 'mulberry' appearance.

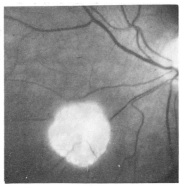

Retinal tumour in tuberous sclerosis.

Von Hippel–Lindau's disease

Haemangioblastomas affect blood vessels in the brainstem, cerebellum and spinal cord. Tumours of the retinal vessels have enormous feeding and draining vessels and may give rise to haemorrhage and retinal detachment. Small tumours are easily eradicated with photocoagulation but large tumours fail to respond.

Recurrent central nervous system involvement usually leads to death in early middle age.

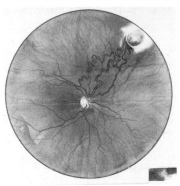

Von Hippel–Lindau's disease.

Rheumatic diseases 28

Many of the diseases coming within the province of the rheumatologist are multisystem disorders in which joint involvement is only a part of the total clinical picture. Ocular manifestations of these rheumatic disorders are often important diagnostic features; not infrequently they constitute the presenting complaint.

Rheumatoid arthritis

Ocular complications of adult rheumatoid arthritis involve either the outer collagenous coats of the eye (sclera, episclera and cornea) or the lacrimal gland.

A typical rheumatoid nodule may develop in the *episclera*. It is painful but resolves without serious sequelae.

Scleritis may take several forms. It may be extremely painful and have a nodular or diffuse appearance or it may be relatively painless and lead to severe thinning of the sclera (scleromalacia perforans).

The *cornea* may be affected by adjacent scleritis or by marginal ulceration which may occur as a separate lesion. Corneal perforation can result.

Management

Topical steroids are of value in the treatment of episcleritis but are generally ineffective in scleritis. They may increase the risk of corneal perforation. Systemic steroids and antimetabolites such as azathioprine are usually effective in controlling scleritis.

Sjögren's syndrome

Keratoconjunctivitis sicca and xerostomia (dry mouth) together constitute the sicca syndrome. Three

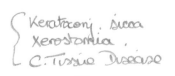

Keratocony. Sicca
Xerostomia,
C. Tissue Disease

out of four patients have an associated connective-tissue disease, the total complex being known as *Sjögren's syndrome*. The connective-tissue disease is usually rheumatoid arthritis but can be systemic lupus erythematosus, polyarteritis nodosa, or scleroderma.

Keratoconjunctivitis sicca occurring as part of Sjögren's syndrome is due to inflammatory and degenerative change in the lacrimal glands. Eventually the gland may be largely replaced by connective tissue. The clinical features and management of kerato-conjunctivitis sicca are discussed in Chapter 9.

Juvenile rheumatoid arthritis (Still's disease)

The ocular manifestations of this disease are quite different from those occurring in the adult form. Children with mono- or pauciarticular arthritis with minimal systemic involvement frequently suffer from iritis which is usually chronic and recurrent. It is frequently bilateral and asymptomatic.

Complications of the iritis are deposition of calcium in the cornea (band keratopathy), cataract and secondary glaucoma.

Management

Children with Still's disease, especially those with minimal joint involvement, should have regular ophthalmological examinations. Iritis is treated with topical steroids and, when necessary, mydriatics but the response is, at best, only partial. Band keratopathy is treated with chelating agents (*see* Chapter 14) and cataract by removal of the lens and anterior vitreous (lensectomy).

Ankylosing spondylitis

Recurrent acute iritis is common in this condition which affects predominantly men. The human leucocyte antigen (HLA B27), which is present in only 5% of the normal population, is found in 96% of patients with ankylosing spondylitis and over 50% of patients with acute iritis. There is also a high incidence of this specific antigen in Reiter's disease, colitic and psoriatic arthropathy.

Reiter's disease

This is predominantly a disease of men and comprises a diagnostic triad of conjunctivitis, urethritis and arthritis. Painless erosions of the oral mucosa are common.

Other ocular complications may occur but these are uncommon. They include episcleritis, keratitis and iritis.

Gonorrhoea must be borne in mind in the differential diagnosis as it may produce the same triad of signs.

[handwritten notes: No₂⁷ Conjunctivitis, Urethritis, Arthritis; also — episcleritis, keratitis, iritis]

Systemic lupus erythematosus (SLE)

This relatively uncommon disease predominantly affects young women. It may affect any system and the clinical picture of the disease varies enormously.

The commonest ocular manifestation of SLE is a characteristic retinopathy with numerous cotton-wool spots and relatively few haemorrhages.

Keratoconjunctivitis sicca may occur in SLE as part of Sjögren's syndrome.

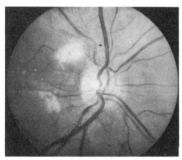

Retinal infarcts in SLE.

Behçet's disease

A disease of unknown aetiology. It is most prevalent in Turkish and Japanese men. There is a high incidence of HLA B5. The clinical triad consists of aphthous stomatitis, genital ulceration and ocular inflammation. Polyarthritis and central nervous system involvement also occur. The latter is usually fatal.

Uveitis is the commonest ocular complication and is often severe and destructive leading eventually to blindness.

[handwritten notes: aphthous stomatitis, Genital ulceration, Uveitis x -severe, Polyarthritis, CNS involvement]

Giant-cell arteritis and polymyalgia rheumatica

There is a close relationship between these two diseases; some patients who present with polymyalgia rheumatica (PMR) go on to develop classical giant-cell (cranial or temporal) arteritis.

The importance of giant-cell arteritis lies in the devastating effect this disease may have upon vision. It is predominantly a disease of the elderly and rarely occurs before the age of 60. Prodromal symptoms include malaise, temporal headache and tenderness, pain on mastication and transient visual loss. Symptoms of PMR may be present and indeed the patient may be under treatment for this condition.

The patient usually presents to the ophthalmologist with sudden loss of vision in one eye (*see* Chapter 2) caused by *ischaemic optic neuropathy*. This is secondary to arteritic involvement of the branches of the ophthalmic artery which supply the anterior part of the optic nerve. The optic nerve is pale and swollen with small haemorrhages on the surface. Much less commonly the central retinal artery itself is occluded leading to infarction of the retina. Ophthalmoplegia may occur but this is uncommon.

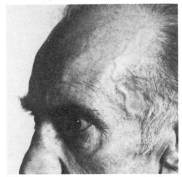
Thickened temporal arteries in giant-cell arteritis.

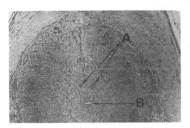
Temporal artery biopsy showing giant cells (A) and tiny residual lumen (B).

Diagnosis

The erythrocyte sedimentation rate is usually elevated, frequently to more than 100 mm/hour. Tenderness and lack of pulsation of one or both temporal arteries is almost diagnostic and histological proof can be obtained with a positive biopsy. A negative biopsy, however, does not rule out the disease.

Management

Corticosteroids must be started immediately the diagnosis is suspected. Initially 60–120 mg of prednisolone (or equivalent) are given daily. The aim of treatment is primarily to prevent loss of vision in the second eye. Recovery of vision in the affected eye is usually very limited.

Corticosteroid therapy is continued at a level sufficient to keep the ESR within the normal range. It is usually continued for at least a year and, even when the steroids are stopped, the patient must be carefully watched for signs of reactivation of the disease.

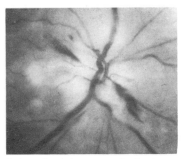
Ischaemic optic neuropathy in giant-cell arteritis.

Polyarteritis nodosa

This disease occasionally causes occlusion of the central retinal artery but more frequently the choroidal circulation is involved. Retinopathy in polyarteritis nodosa may be secondary to associated hypertension but may be caused by a retinal vasculitis with haemorrhage, exudate and cotton-wool spots.

Polyarteritis may also produce multiple cranial nerve palsies and other neurological manifestations including visual field defects and Horner's syndrome.

Gout

There is an association between gout and scleritis. The latter is often of sudden onset, is very painful, and may precede or accompany joint involvement.

Infectious and granulomatous disease

29

The eye is involved in a wide variety of systemic infections, the ocular features of which are often characteristic of the disease. Also included in this chapter are the ocular manifestations of sarcoidosis, a granulomatous disease of unknown aetiology.

Bacterial disease

Septicaemia

The eye is not commonly involved in bacterial septicaemia though endophthalmitis or orbital cellulitis may develop. In *subacute bacterial endocarditis* characteristic flame-shaped retinal haemorrhages with white centres (*Roth spots*) are seen.

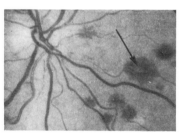

Roth spot.

Syphilis

New cases of *congenital* syphilis are now rare, but patients from the pre-antibiotic era are still seen bearing the hallmark of the disease, *interstitial keratitis*. Inflammation of the cornea in childhood has left these individuals with scarred corneas through which run empty 'ghost' blood vessels. These are visible on slit-lamp examination. Vision may remain at reasonable levels but severely affected cases require keratoplasty. Patients with congenital syphilis may also have a *pigmentary 'salt and pepper' retinopathy* and *optic atrophy*.

Most newly *acquired* cases of syphilis occur in male homosexuals. The secondary stage of the disease may present as uveitis or, less frequently, retinitis, often associated with a typical skin rash.

The majority of patients with tertiary syphilis also come from the pre-antibiotic era. *Argyll Robertson*

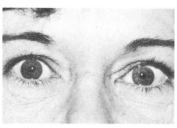

Argyll Robertson pupils.

pupils (*see* Chapter 15) indicate tabes dorsalis. Meningovascular syphilis is seldom seen now but at one time was an important cause of optic atrophy and blindness.

Gonorrhoea

The gonococcus used to be a common cause of *ophthalmia neonatorum*—ocular infection occurring during passage of the infant through the birth canal. Infection can produce a severe purulent conjunctivitis with marked lid swelling and a high risk of corneal perforation.

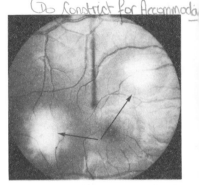

Choroidal tubercles (arrowed). Dark line is fixation target.

Tuberculosis

Prior to effective chemotherapy tuberculosis was a major cause of severe *uveitis and phlyctenular* disease of the cornea. Miliary involvement of the choroid is occasionally seen.

Leprosy

Leprosy is an important cause of blindness in the underdeveloped world. Facial palsy and its complications are common in all forms of the disease and chronic uveitis and secondary cataract occur in lepromatous leprosy.

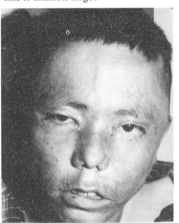

Facial palsy in leprosy.

Chlamydial infection

Chlamydia are obligate intracellular organisms with some characteristics of both bacteria and viruses. *Chlamydia trachomatis* is the agent responsible for one of the commonest causes of blindness in the world— trachoma. This chronic follicular conjunctivitis, which is endemic in many areas of the underdeveloped world, is discussed in Chapter 6.

The same organism is responsible for an acute, but less serious form of conjunctivitis in the developed world. This is known as *inclusion conjunctivitis* because of the presence of inclusion bodies which may be seen in the cells scraped from the infected conjunctiva. The organism may infect the uterine cervix and rectum and the disease is transmitted sexually in young adults or during birth when it causes *ophthalmia neonatorum*.

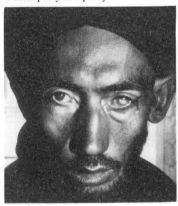

Trachomatous scarring of the cornea.

Viral infections

Herpes zoster

Reactivation of latent varicella-zoster virus within the geniculate ganglion causes herpes zoster opthalmicus if the first division of the fifth cranial nerve is involved. The virus spreads peripherally along the sensory nerve causing a painful, unilateral vesicular eruption over the forehead, upper eyelid and nose. It lasts for several weeks and heals leaving pitted scars. If the tip of the nose is spared (nasociliary nerve) the eye is less likely to be involved.

Conjunctivitis is common but seldom significant. Corneal changes range from a mild neurotrophic *keratitis* with punctate epithelial erosions and the formation of dendritic figures to total loss of sensation and severe corneal scarring. *Anterior uveitis* is common and there may be associated *secondary glaucoma* (from inflammation of the trabecular meshwork). Less common complications are scleritis, optic neuritis and ocular motor nerve palsies.

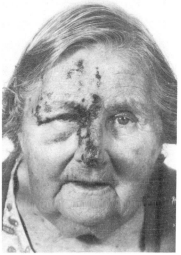
Herpes zoster ophthalmicus.

Management

Early treatment of the vesicular rash with a solution of idoxuridine in dimethyl sulphoxide reduces the severity of post-herpetic neuralgia. Antibiotic sprays are helpful in reducing secondary infection of the skin. Topical steroids are invaluable in controlling inflammatory disease of the anterior segment of the eye but if their use is prolonged, and this is often necessary, the intraocular pressure must be carefully monitored

Chickenpox, caused by the identical varicella virus, seldom involves the eye though vesicles may occur on the conjunctiva and lid margins.

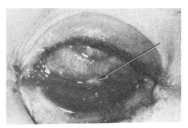
Conjunctival vesicle in chickenpox.

Herpes simplex

Ocular disease is caused by the type 1 virus which is also responsible for lesions of the skin, mucous membranes and brain. The *primary* infection may cause a vesicular eruption around the lids and a follicular conjunctivitis with no, or minimal, corneal involvement. The virus is thought to then remain latent, either in the posterior root ganglion of the fifth nerve or possibly within the lacrimal gland, until triggered to cause recurrent ocular disease.

- infected in infancy – by being kissed by adults.
Labial/Eye = 50/1.
offers slight protection against eye infection.

Corneal involvement is a cause of the acute red eye (*see* Chapter 7) but the disease may become chronic and result in severe scarring and loss of vision. Involvement of the deeper layers of the cornea is frequently accompanied by uveitis and secondary glaucoma. Metaherpetic keratitis.

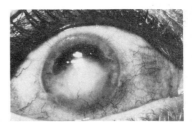

Severe corneal scarring from herpes simplex.

Cytomegalovirus

Congenital infection, by transfer of the virus across the placenta, causes hepatosplenomegaly, microcephaly (with mental retardation and cerebral calcification) and inflammation of the choroid and retina. *Acquired infection* rarely causes serious ocular disease but in immune-deficient individuals, such as those patients on immunosuppressive treatment or suffering from the acquired immune deficiency syndrome (AIDS) an active chorioretinitis resulting in loss of vision may occur.

Rubella

Fetal infection with the rubella virus during the first trimester causes widespread systemic abnormalities, particularly of the cardiovascular system and special senses. The ocular manifestations are considered in Chapter 32. The congenital rubella syndrome is now preventable since the introduction of effective vaccines and should in time become a rare occurrence.

Measles

Photophobia and mild conjunctivitis occur in this acute infectious disease but serious ocular sequelae are rare in the developed world. However, in areas of the world where malnutrition is widespread the measles virus is a significant cause of blindness through corneal ulceration and scarring.

Fungal disease

Fungal infections of the eye are uncommon but are being seen with increasing frequency. This is due to a number of factors, particularly those which reduce host resistance and allow opportunistic infections to develop. The widespread use of topical steroids, immunosuppression following transplant surgery and the acquired immune deficiency syndrome (AIDS) are examples.

Candida

This is the most common ocular fungal pathogen. The serious ocular manifestations are keratitis and endophthalmitis. The latter is seen most frequently among drug addicts who inject substances intravenously. Fluffy yellow-white lesions are seen in the vitreous or on the retinal surface and the associated uveitis is responsible for the presenting symptoms which include blurring of vision, redness and pain. Ocular morbidity is high in spite of systemic treatment with antifungal agents such as 5-fluorocytosine and amphotericin B.

Many other fungal species including aspergillus and fusarium cause ocular disease similar to candida.

Histoplasmosis, a fungal disease endemic in the southern United States, produces a specific clinical picture within the eye with visual loss resulting from macular scarring.

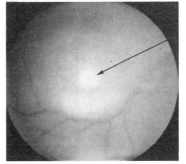

Candida endophthalmitis—fungal mass on surface of retina.

Protozoan disease

Toxoplasmosis

Acquired disease, caused by the protozoon, *Toxoplasma gondii*, is common. In some areas 50% of the population over the age of 50 years show immunological evidence of infection. It seldom, however, causes significant clinical illness and ocular involvement in the acquired disease is rare.

Congenital toxoplasmosis has a predilection for the central nervous system resulting in the characteristic triad of convulsions, intracranial calcification and chorioretinitis. Ocular involvement, which may be the only manifestation of the disease, is the commonest cause of posterior uveitis and is particularly prevalent in Negroes. The toxoplasma dye test is occasionally helpful but 20% of normal adults have a positive dye test titre of 1 : 8. A rising titre is usually only found in acquired infection.

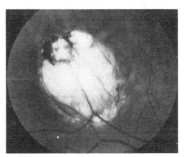

Congenital toxoplasmosis scar.

Helminthic diseases

The eye may be affected by tapeworm larvae in *cysticercosis (Taenia solium)* and *hydatid disease (Echinococcus granulosus)*. In the former the larvae cause severe intraocular inflammation; in hydatid disease orbital cysts may cause proptosis.

Nematode infestation is seen in *toxocariasis* (*see* Chapter 32) and *onchocerciasis*. The latter disease, also known as 'river blindness' is a major cause of blindness in several parts of the world (*see* Chapter 6).

Sarcoidosis

Sarcoidosis is a multisystem granulomatous disorder of unknown cause which frequently affects the eyes.

The most common ocular manifestation is *uveitis*. Acute anterior uveitis occurs in the younger age group, more often in women, and may be associated with erythema nodosum and bilateral hilar lymphadenopathy. Chronic anterior uveitis occurs in older patients and giant 'mutton fat' keratic precipitates are often seen.

Inflammation of the posterior part of the eye may take the form of *choroidal nodules*, *retinal vasculitis* and *vitreous ('snowball') opacities*.

Papilloedema may be secondary to posterior uveitis or be a manifestation of neurosarcoidosis. *Facial palsy* is the commonest neurological presentation.

Sarcoid follicles are occasionally seen in the *conjunctiva*. They cause minimal symptoms but are easy to biopsy and may confirm the diagnosis. *Kerato-conjunctivitis sicca* occurs in chronic persistent sarcoidosis and is often accompanied by enlargement of the lacrimal glands.

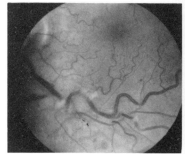

Retinal vasculitis in sarcoidosis.

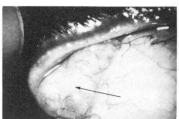

Enlargement of the lacrimal gland.

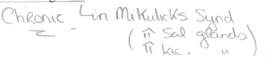

[handwritten annotation:] Chronic → in Mikulicks Synd (↑ Sal glands) (↑ Lac. glands)

Blood disorders

30

Anaemia

The commonest finding in anaemia is pallor of the tarsal conjunctiva. Retinal haemorrhages may be seen and some have white centres (Roth spots). Retinal infarcts and oedema may also be present. This retinopathy rarely occurs unless the haemoglobin levels are less than 50% of normal and other factors such as platelet deficiency and hypoxic capillary damage are probably involved.

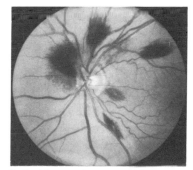

Retinal haemorrhages.

Acute blood loss

Acute blood loss, particularly from gastrointestinal haemorrhage in a patient already suffering from chronic iron-deficiency anaemia, can produce profound visual loss often several days later. The optic discs are pale and swollen, showing the features of ischaemic optic neuropathy. The end result may be blindness with optic atrophy, but recovery of vision can occur.

Macrocytic (pernicious) anaemia

Pernicious anaemia is due to vitamin B_{12} deficiency. In addition to anaemic retinopathy, as described above, optic neuropathy may occur. There is loss of visual acuity and colour vision, in particular to red and green, is defective. A centrocaecal scotoma (an area involving fixation and the blind spot) can be demonstrated. The condition is similar to tobacco/alcohol amblyopia and is related to a deficiency of hydroxycobalamin. Periodic intra-muscular injection of hydroxocobalamin is required.

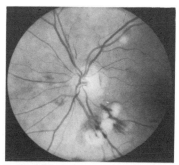

Retinal infarcts and haemorrhages in pernicious anaemia.

Sickle-cell disease

This is a group of genetic disorders in which sickle haemoglobin (HbS) replaces normal, adult haemoglobin (HbA). The red blood corpuscles become deformed ('sickle') when the oxygen tension is low. Ocular changes occur, especially in the peripheral retina. Both homozygous sickle-cell anaemia (SS) and sickle-cell haemoglobin C (SC) disease affect the eye.

Characteristic ocular manifestations of sickle-cell disease include:

1. Vascular proliferations from the peripheral retina into the vitreous ('sea fans').

2. Choroidal infarction with scattering of the overlying pigment (black 'sunburst' spots).

Eventually proliferative retinopathy, similar to that seen in diabetes, may occur with detachment of the retina and, frequently, secondary glaucoma.

The role of photocoagulation is less certain than in diabetes but similar surgical techniques are required to correct retinal detachment.

Polycythaemia

Polycythaemia from any cause results in increased blood viscosity. This is responsible for the ocular manifestations which include dilatation of the conjunctival and iris vessels and engorgement of the retinal veins. The latter is associated with retinal haemorrhages and optic disc oedema; thrombosis of the central retinal vein may supervene. Occlusion of the central retinal artery also occurs.

Other blood disorders causing high viscosity (e.g. macroglobulinaemia) can produce a similar picture.

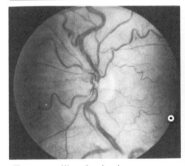

Tortuous dilated veins in polycythaemia.

Leukaemia

The retinopathy of leukaemia is due in part to infiltration of the retinal tissues with immature white cells but also to the associated anaemia

Flame-shaped haemorrhages with a white centre (Roth spots) and cotton-wool spots are common in acute leukaemia and are frequently accompanied by distension of the retinal veins and arterioles. Haemorrhage may also occur into the eyelids and subconjunctivally.

Subconjunctival lymphomas, presenting as painless fleshy tumours on the globe or inner aspect of the eyelid occur in lymphatic leukaemia. Leukaemic infiltration of the optic nerve is rare but can cause blindness.

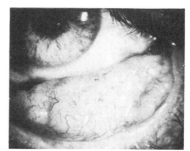

Subconjunctival lymphoma.

Thrombocytopenia

Platelet deficiency diseases cause a retinopathy, similar to that of severe anaemia, with retinal haemorrhages, oedema and cotton-wool spots. Bleeding from iris vessels may cause recurrent hyphaemas.

Skin and mucous membrane disorders

31

Acne rosacea

Acne rosacea is a chronic acneiform eruption which involves the face. There is cutaneous erythema and inflammation of the pilosebaceous follicles. It occurs more frequently in women and usually between the ages of 30 and 50 years.

Ocular manifestations include blepharoconjunctivitis and recurrent chalazia. A small percentage of patients develop rosacea keratitis in which there is progressive vascularization and scarring of the cornea.

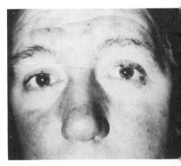

Acne rosacea.

Management

Systemic tetracycline therapy is effective in reducing the severity of the ocular complications. Topical steroids may be necessary to control corneal disease; occasionally corneal grafting is necessary.

Psoriasis

This common, chronic disorder of the skin is characterized by slightly raised erythematous patches covered by whitish or silver scales. Ocular complications include blepharoconjunctivitis and vascular infiltration of the cornea. Patients with psoriatic arthropathy may develop uveitis (*see* Chapter 28).

154

Eczema

Eczema is a descriptive term which implies a skin reaction with an allergic mechanism. Signs and symptoms include erythema, vesicle formation, oozing, crusting, thickening and itching.

A non-specific type of eczema affecting the eyelids may occur in a variety of generalized skin disorders such as atopic dermatitis, seborrheic dermatitis, and psoriasis.

occasionally ⟶ presenile Cataract

Allergic oedema

Acute swelling of the eyelids may occur as part of a generalized allergic reaction or have a local cause. There is usually an atopic or type I anaphylactic hypersensitivity. General causes include angioneurotic oedema and drug reactions; insect bites are a common local cause.

Management

The laxity of the eyelid tissues allows gross swelling to occur which may alarm the patient. Reassurance is all that is required in the absence of serious systemic involvement such as glottal oedema.

Pemphigus

Pemphigus is characterized by the formation of intraepidermal bullae which arise in apparently normal skin and mucous membrane. Conjunctival involvement may lead to the formation of symblepharon (adhesions between tarsal and bulbar conjunctiva). Distortion of the lids and lashes may cause corneal damage.

Benign mucous membrane pemphigoid

In this condition the bullae are submucosal. It affects predominantly the elderly and the disease may be limited to the conjunctiva. Involvement of other mucosa may lead to strictures of the oesophagus, urethra, vagina and anus.

Initially the disease may present as a chronic unilateral recurrent conjunctivitis but eventually it becomes bilateral with conjunctival scarring and symblepharon formation. Corneal damage occurs secondary to dryness and entropion and the resulting ulceration and scarring frequently lead to blindness. In this sense the disease is not 'benign'; pemphigus, on the other hand, rarely leads to blindness.

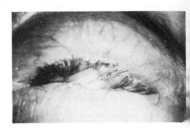

Entropion and trichiasis in mucous membrane pemphigoid.

Management

There is no effective treatment but tear substitutes and the correction of lid deformities help minimize corneal damage. Therapeutic contact lenses are occasionally useful.

Erythema multiforme

Erythema multiforme is a disease of unknown aetiology in which prodromal symptoms of malaise, myalgia and fever are followed by the development of inflammatory skin lesions. A wide variety of agents have been incriminated as precipitating factors including bacteria, viruses and drugs, especially sulphonamides.

The eye is most commonly involved in the severe bullous form of the disease in which mucous membrane is involved—the Stevens–Johnson syndrome. This affects predominantly children and young adults.

Ocular complications vary from mild conjunctivitis to severe conjunctival scarring with symblepharon formation, lid deformity, dryness and corneal ulceration.

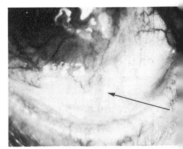

Conjunctival scarring in Stevens–Johnson syndrome.

Management

Local and systemic steroids may limit the degree of conjunctival scarring. Topical antibiotics are required to combat secondary infection. Tear substitutes and surgical correction of lid deformities are often necessary to prevent chronic corneal damage.

Paediatric disorders 32

The commonest eye disorders in childhood are squint and obstruction of the nasolacrimal duct. These have been considered in Part I. Other disorders may present as an abnormal appearance of the eye, e.g. a white pupil or enlarged globe, or they may be recognized as part of a wider paediatric problem. For convenience they are all considered in this chapter though in some conditions there may be no systemic implications.

The white pupil (leukocoria)

The normal pupil is black and a white pupillary reflex indicates serious eye disease. The mother is usually the first person to notice this and should always be believed. Urgent assessment by an ophthalmologist is required.

The major causes of this condition are :

Congenital cataract
Retinoblastoma
Retrolental fibroplasia

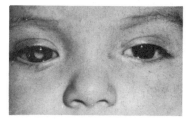

Leukocoria.

Congenital cataract

The majority of congenital cataracts are familial. Other causes include rubella, galactosaemia and hypocalcaemia.

Some congenital cataracts cause little visual impairment but others are so dense that early surgical removal is required in order to allow normal development of vision. The optical correction of aphakia in young infants is difficult as very high

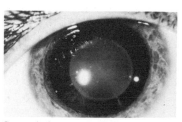

Congenital cataract—central opacity.

degrees of hypermetropia are encountered. However, soft contact lenses can be successfully used, even in the very young, and the visual results of bilateral cataract extraction are often excellent.

The treatment of unilateral cataract is less satisfactory unless the surgery is carried out at a very early stage and followed by energetic treatment to prevent amblyopia.

Retinoblastoma

This rare tumour affects about 1 in 25 000 infants. The commonest presenting feature in infancy is a white pupil or squint though in later childhood it may be uveitis. One or both eyes can be affected. Ten per cent are hereditary (dominant), the remainder sporadic.

Extensive involvement of the eye requires enucleation but smaller tumours may be destroyed by radiation or cryotherapy with the preservation of useful vision. Very careful follow-up and genetic counselling are necessary.

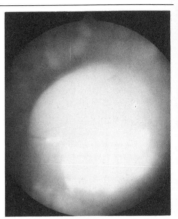

Retinoblastoma—white mass in fundus.

Retrolental fibroplasia

Vascularization of the fetal retina is not complete until term. Thus in premature babies the peripheral retina is avascular. Those vessels which are present are very sensitive to oxygen levels in the blood and if this is too high the terminal branches may constrict. In the early stages this is reversible and orderly development continues when conditions return to normal.

However, in severe cases new vessels proliferate from the sites of constriction into the vitreous and become covered in fibrous tissue to form a fibrovascular membrane behind the lens which contracts causing retinal detachment. The disease is usually bilateral and may result in total blindness.

Treatment of the established condition is extremely difficult and prevention is of the utmost importance. This is possible by careful monitoring of the blood oxygen levels of premature infants who require oxygen therapy. A delicate balance has to be struck between the respiratory requirements and the risk of damage to the eyes.

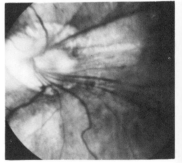

Retinal traction in retrolental fibroplasia.

Congenital glaucoma (buphthalmos)

Glaucoma in childhood is uncommon. The cause is usually a developmental abnormality of the angle of the anterior chamber which impedes aqueous drainage. The sclera and cornea of the infant eye are much less rigid than in the adult and the eye distends as a result of raised intraocular pressure (buphthalmos means ox eye). The presenting clinical features, apart from enlargement of the globe, are haziness of the cornea due to oedema, watering and photophobia. Usually both eyes are affected.

Treatment of this condition is surgical. The abnormal tissue overlying the drainage angle is divided by a knife and this procedure, called goniotomy, allows the restoration of normal aqueous drainage. The globe, however, remains large in spite of normalization of the intraocular pressure.

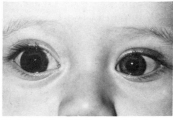

Unilateral buphthalmos—right eye.

Rubella

Maternal infection within the first 3 months of fetal life can cause serious cardiac, auditory and ocular complications.

The ocular complications include :

1. *Cataract*
2. *Microphthalmos*
3. *Glaucoma*
4. *Retinopathy*
5. *Uveitis*

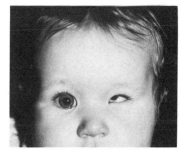

Microphthalmos in rubella syndrome.

They may occur separately or together. The retinopathy is comparatively benign but the first 3 features, which can affect one or both eyes, result in severely limited vision.

Toxocara

Puppies are frequently infected with nematodes and the eggs are passed in faeces. Contamination of fingers may result in small children ingesting the larvae of

Toxocara canis which pass into the circulation and occasionally lodge in the eye to produce a retinal granuloma and uveitis. The granuloma usually develops in the macular area resulting in loss of central vision and frequently development of a squint.

Clinically it may be difficult to differentiate a toxocara granuloma (which contains the larva) from a retinoblastoma. There is no treatment for the condition and regular worming of household pets, especially puppies, is the best preventive measure.

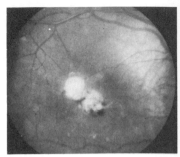

Toxocara granuloma at macula.

Down's syndrome

This common genetic abnormality is due to trisomy of chromosome 21.

The ophthalmic features of this condition include:

1. A *mongoloid* slant of the palpebral fissures giving the syndrome its original name of mongolism.
2. *Epicanthic folds.*
3. *Blepharitis.* This is often severe with extensive crusting of the lid margins.
4. *Refractive errors.* High myopia is frequently encountered.
5. *Squint* is common and it may be difficult to prevent amblyopia as occlusion of the good eye may not be tolerated by the child.
6. *Cataract* and *keratoconus* also occur in association with Down's syndrome but these are not common. Pale patches on the iris (*Brushfield's spots*) are prominent in children with Down's syndrome though they also occur in normal people.

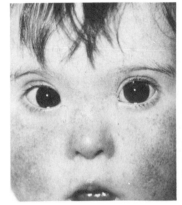

Down's syndrome.

Hydrocephalus

Raised intracranial pressure occurring before fusion of the sutures of the vault of the skull results in enlargement of the head and not papilloedema. The characteristic ocular sign of hydrocephalus is conjugate deviation of the eyes downward (the sign of the setting sun) but vision is mainly at risk from acute angulation of the optic nerves resulting from the change in shape of the skull.

Hydrocephalus is now preventable by operations designed to shunt cerebrospinal fluid from the ventricles to the venous side of the circulation but repeated surgery can damage the optic radiations.

Marfan's syndrome

The clinical features of this disorder, which is inherited as a dominant trait, are due to mesodermal hypoplasia. The outstanding ocular manifestation is *subluxation* (partial displacement) or *dislocation* of the lens.

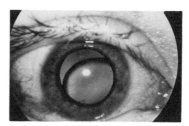

Subluxated lens in Marfan's syndrome.

This may cause severe visual difficulties if the edge of the lens coincides with the visual axis. A choice has to be made between correcting the myopic astigmatism in the phakic portion of the pupil or the aphakic vision where the lens is absent. Lens extraction in this condition is very difficult and complications are frequent.

A dislocated lens may cause secondary glaucoma by obstructing the passage of aqueous through the pupil. Other complications include chronic glaucoma and retinal detachment.

Dislocation of the lens also occurs in homocystinuria.

Part 3

Ophthalmic investigations and treatment

Diagnostic tests 33

Special diagnostic tests are now employed routinely in the investigation of a wide variety of ocular diseases. These include :

Fluorescein angiography
Ultrasonography
Computerized tomography
Electrodiagnosis

Fluorescein angiography

Detailed examination of the retinal circulation is facilitated by the use of a fluorescent dye. A small bolus of sodium fluorescein is injected into an antecubital vein and photographs of the fundus of the eye are taken in rapid sequence by a retinal camera incorporating filters which exclude non-fluorescent light.

The choroidal circulation fills rapidly but is seen only as a diffuse blush in the healthy eye. There is leakage of dye from the choroidal capillaries but this is masked by the overlying retinal pigment epithelium. In contrast, fluorescein does not escape from the normal retinal circulation. Filling of the retinal arterioles is almost instantaneous while that of the retinal veins is slower and laminar due to delayed return from the peripheral retina.

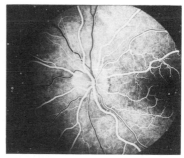

Fluorescein angiogram—early filling of veins.

Fluorescein angiography is valuable in the assessment of retinal vascular disease, such as diabetic retinopathy, when leaking vessels, capillary closure and retinal neovascularization may be identified. Other uses include the investigation of macular disease and the differential diagnosis of optic disc swelling and fundus tumours.

Ultrasonography

Ultrasound biometry of the eye is employed in the preoperative assessment of the cataract patient in whom intraocular lens implantation is planned. The axial length of the eye is measured using an *A-scan* and the required power of the lens is calculated from this and the radius of curvature of the cornea.

The *B-scan* produces a cross-section 'picture' of the eye and retro-ocular space which can be recorded from the oscilloscope screen on polaroid film. This is of great value in assessing the posterior segment of the eye when examination of the fundus is precluded by a dense cataract or vitreous haemorrhage. Retinal detachment and choroidal tumour can be readily diagnosed. Orbital tumours may be detected by ultrasonography but x-ray studies are generally more satisfactory.

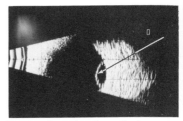

B-scan of eye showing retinal detachment (arrowed).

Computerized tomography

The high resolution of current CT scanners allows the main structures of the eye and orbit to be clearly visualized. It is an invaluable tool in the investigation of orbital disease and in the identification of intracranial causes of optic atrophy, papilloedema and visual field loss.

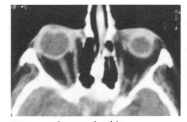

CT scan of eye and orbit.

Electrodiagnosis

1. The electro-oculogram (EOG)

This records the resting potential of the retina through electrodes placed on the skin at the inner and outer canthus of each eye. This potential changes with the level of retinal illumination and depends on the health of the retinal photoreceptors and their pigments, the pigment epithelium and the choroid. An abnormal EOG is found in retinitis pigmentosa, vitamin A deficiency and retinal detachment.

2. The electroretinogram (ERG)

This records the retinal response to a flash and indicates the functional state of all layers of the retina excluding the ganglion cell layer. The ERG is recorded using an active electrode on the cornea and a reference electrode on the forehead. By using coloured or flickering flashes it is possible to distinguish between cone and rod function. Uses include the detection of the early stages of retinitis pigmentosa, hereditary macular degeneration, colour blindness and night blindness. Electroretinography also allows functional assessment of the retina in an eye with a dense cataract or vitreous haemorrhage.

3. The visually-evoked response (VER)

This is the visually-evoked response of the EEG recorded at the occipital pole. The stimulus may be a flash or a pattern of checks or gratings. If the EOG and ERG are normal an abnormal VER indicates an organic lesion of the visual pathway between and including the retinal ganglion cells and the visual cortex. It is particularly valuable in the diagnosis of demyelination of nerve fibres in the CNS, when there is delayed conduction, and in differentiating organic and functional causes of poor vision in suspected hysteria and malingering.

Optical aids

Refractive errors can be corrected by either spectacle lenses or contact lenses. They provide a focused image on the retina and any magnification or minification is incidental. If magnification is required to improve vision in the diseased eye then low vision aids are prescribed.

Spectacle lenses

These may be manufactured to incorporate one or more focal powers.

Single focus lenses

These are commonly prescribed for the correction of myopia and, as reading glasses, for the correction of presbyopia.

Multifocal lenses

Bifocal lenses are commonly worn by the middle-aged and elderly to correct both distance and near vision with one pair of spectacles.

Trifocals increase the range by incorporating an intermediate segment.

Variable focus lenses attempt to produce focused vision at all distances by a gradual change in the focal power of the lens from top to bottom. This is achieved at the expense of some peripheral distortion.

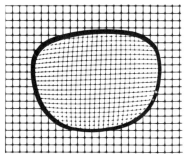

Myopic lens.

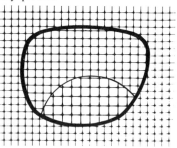

Hypermetropic bifocal lens.

Spectacle lenses can be made of glass, toughened glass or plastic. Various tints and anti-reflective coatings may be incorporated; these are nearly always for the patient's comfort or to satisfy his or her vanity and rarely for any medical reason.

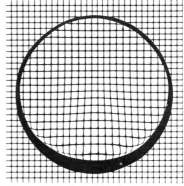

Hypermetropic variable focus lens.

Contact lenses

Contact lenses are worn on the surface of the eye and are usually prescribed for the correction of refractive errors. Occasionally they are used therapeutically to protect the corneal surface or cosmetically to hide an unsightly eye.

There are two main types of contact lens in common use:

Hard contact lenses

These are made of polymethylmethacrylate and are smaller than the corneal diameter. They float on the cornea on a film of tears and will correct the majority of refractive errors including moderate degrees of astigmatism. The main disadvantage with this type of lens is that tolerance is limited. If the lenses are worn for too long (the normal wearing time is up to about 18 hours) then the cornea shows signs of oxygen deprivation and the eye becomes painful with blurred vision.

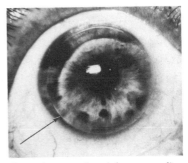

Corneal contact lens (edge arrowed).

Soft contact lenses

These are made of hydrophilic polymers and contain a high percentage of water. They overlap the corneal margin and fit flush with the corneal surface; this ability of the lens to mould limits the amount of corneal astigmatism that can be corrected.

The major advantage of soft contact lenses lies in the ease with which they can be worn. Oxygen penetration is high and they may be worn for long periods without discomfort. However, sterilization is more critical than with hard lenses and contamination may lead to serious ocular infection.

Lenses made of *gas-permeable* material are available which incorporate some of the features of both hard and soft lenses.

Use of contact lenses

Visual

1. MYOPIA

Low and moderate degrees of myopia are satisfactorily corrected by both types of contact lens. Visually there is little advantage over spectacles and the main motivation is often cosmetic though they are advantageous in many sports. Vision in <u>high myopia</u> is often considerably improved by a contact lens.

2. ASTIGMATISM

Moderate degrees of <u>regular astigmatism</u> can be corrected with <u>either contact lenses or spectacles</u>. However conditions giving rise to *irregular astigmatism* (especially keratoconus) can <u>often only</u> be satisfactorily corrected <u>with contact lenses</u>.

3. APHAKIA

Contact lenses have <u>distinct advantages</u> over spectacles in the correction of aphakia (*see* Chapter 35).

- image 10% Magnification
- V. acuity usually good.
- No peripheral Distortions.

Therapeutic

Thin soft contact lenses ('bandage lenses') are used to relieve ocular discomfort caused by loss of corneal epithelium in recurrent corneal abrasion (*see* Chapter 21) and bullous keratopathy (chronic oedema of the cornea). They are also used to prevent damage to the cornea from trichiasis and to allow healing of indolent corneal ulcers. ⌐ misalignment of the eyelashes.

Cosmetic

Shrunken and disorganized (phthisical) eyes can be hidden by acrylic shells painted to match the fellow eye. These cover the entire anterior segment of the eye. Dense corneal scars and iris defects can be camouflaged by the use of coloured soft lenses with a clear or black central 'pupil' as required.

Low vision aids

These are prescribed for patients with central visual defects, usually the result of macular disease. There are no satisfactory optical aids for the correction of visual field defects such as homonymous hemianopia.

The provision of 'extra strong' reading glasses may allow the patient with low visual acuity to hold print nearer to the eye so allowing some enlargement of the text.

True magnification can be provided in a variety of ways:

1. MAGNIFYING LENSES

These are held or positioned close to the print in order the produce a magnified image. These magnifying lenses are used in conjunction with reading glasses if worn.

2. TELESCOPIC AIDS

Miniaturized Galilean telescopes may be hand held for distance vision (e.g. reading street signs) or incorporated into a spectacle frame for reading.

3. CLOSED CIRCUIT TELEVISION

A television camera provides variable magnification of text which can be viewed on a monitor.

The higher the degree of magnification obtained with an aid the smaller the field of vision. Other factors limiting the usefulness of low vision aids include the size of the central scotoma, the amount of distortion present and the motivation of the patient.

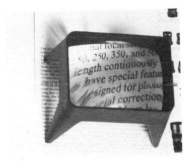

Magnifying glass.

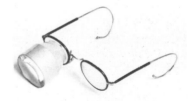

Telescopic spectacles.

Incision and curettage of Meibomian cyst

Topical anaesthesia is applied to the conjunctiva and the lid infiltrated with lignocaine.

The area of the lid containing the cyst is held in a clamp and the cyst is opened through its conjunctival surface by an incision at right angles to the lid margin (to avoid cutting across adjacent Meibomian glands). The contents of the cyst are removed with a small curette. A fibrous chalazion may need to be excised.

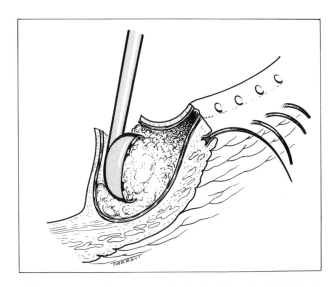

Tarsorrhaphy

The upper and lower lid margins can be joined laterally or centrally. Local anaesthesia is normally employed.

A thin strip of skin is removed from the lid margins, just posterior to the lashes, and the areas are apposed with sutures until healing has taken place in about ten days.

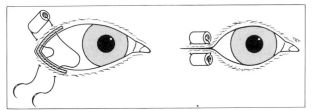

- Use tubes to ↑ the surface area of contact.
→ > area over which healing (by 2° intention) will occur.

Senile ectropion

The lower lid is tightened by shortening its length. A wedge of conjunctiva and tarsal plate is removed and a triangle of skin and muscle is excised to bring the lid into its correct position.

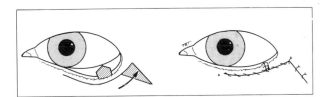

Senile entropion

There are many different operations for the correction of this condition. The common aim is to prevent the orbicularis muscle riding up over the anterior surface of the tarsal plate (so inverting the lower lid); this can be achieved either by muscle excision or the creation of scar tissue. Shortening of the tarsal plate may also be employed.

Ptosis

Operations to correct ptosis are planned depending on the degree of action of the levator palpebrae superioris.

General anaesthesia is normally employed. The operation shown below entails exposure of the levator muscle, resection of a predetermined length and resuturing of the muscle end to the tarsal plate.

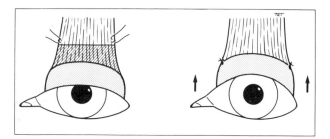

Squint

Surgical correction aims to place the eyes in the normal position and allow full movement. Overactive muscles are weakened by recession in which the original insertion is moved posteriorly; weak muscles are strengthened by resection.

The operation shown here shows the medial rectus muscle being recessed and the lateral rectus muscle resected in order to correct a convergent deviation.

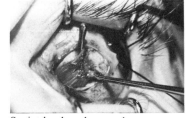

Squint hook under muscle.

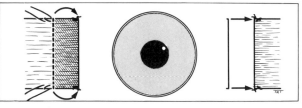

Lateral rectus.   Medial rectus.

Retinal detachment

The fundamental aim in treating primary retinal detachment is to seal the hole in the retina.

This is achieved by indenting the sclera to allow apposition of retina and choroid at the site of the hole. A permanent adhesion is then formed by inducing an inflammatory reaction between the two tissues by means of cryotherapy which is applied through the sclera.

Indentation is achieved by suturing a piece of silicone rubber sponge onto the sclera.

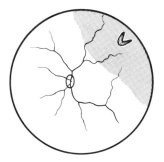
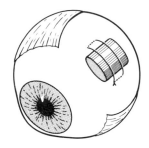
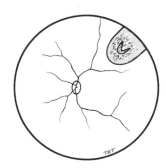

Corneal graft (keratoplasty)

The diseased area of the patient's cornea is trephined out and a similar sized 'button' of healthy cornea taken from a donor eye is sutured in place.

The high success rate of this operation is due to the avascular nature of the tissue but graft rejection can occur.

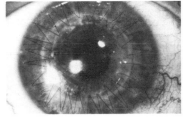

Corneal graft with continuous nylon suture.

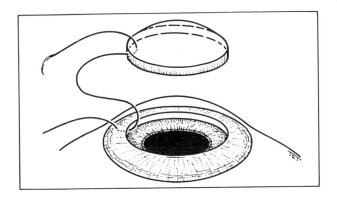

Cataract

Cataract extraction is one of the most successful of all operations and in ophthalmic practice is the most frequently performed.

The lens can be detached from its suspensory ligament (zonule) and removed completely (*intracapsular extraction*) or the anterior capsule, lens nucleus and cortex can be removed leaving the posterior capsule and zonule intact (*extracapsular extraction*). The eye is entered by an incision through the upper edge of the cornea. During *intracapsular extraction* the suspensory ligament is digested by injection of alpha-chymotrypsin solution into the posterior chamber allowing the lens to be easily removed after 2 or 3 minutes with the aid of forceps or a cryoprobe.

In *extracapsular extraction* the anterior capsule is carefully removed, the hard nucleus is expressed from the eye and the remaining cortex removed by suction and irrigation.

The incision is then sutured with fine silk or monofilament nylon sutures to provide tight closure of the eye.

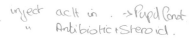

inject aclt in . → Pupil Const
     "   Antibiotic + Steroid.

The type of cataract extraction employed depends on a variety of factors including the type of intraocular lens that may be inserted and the surgeon's own preference for a particular technique. The success rate with intra- and extracapsular extraction is high.

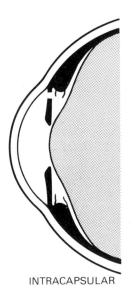
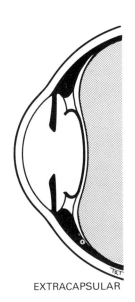

INTRACAPSULAR   EXTRACAPSULAR

Correction of aphakia

Removal of the cystalline lens leaves the emmetropic eye grossly hypermetropic.

This can be corrected with spectacles but the image size is increased by about 30%. This type of correction gives excellent visual acuity but the powerful lens induces various peripheral distortions which many patients find unacceptable. In addition, the degree of magnification is such that fusion of the images of each eye is impossible unless both eyes are aphakic.

Contact lenses may also be used to correct aphakia. Less magnification is produced (10%), visual acuity is usually good and peripheral distortions are eliminated. The degree of magnification is small enough to allow fusion if the other eye is phakic. However, some patients are unable to tolerate a contact lens and others, especially the elderly, have great difficulty in handling them.

A third method of correcting the refractive error is by the insertion of an *intraocular lens* either at the time of extraction or as a secondary procedure. The image size is virtually normal. The strength of the intraocular lens required can be calculated preoperatively from measurements of the axial length of the eye (by ultrasonography) and the curvature of the cornea. This is now a popular method of correcting aphakia, especially in the elderly patient. The lenses which are made of polymethylmethacrylate may be:

1. Inserted entirely anterior to the iris (*anterior chamber lens*).

2. Held in place by loops passing in front and behind the iris through the pupil (*iris-clip lens*).

3. Inserted between the iris and posterior capusule (*posterior chamber lens*).

The last method is now widely employed.

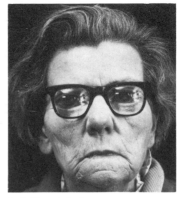
Aphakic spectacles.

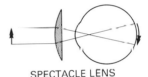
SPECTACLE LENS

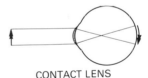
CONTACT LENS

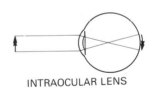
INTRAOCULAR LENS

Iris-clip intraocular lens.

Glaucoma

In *acute glaucoma* aqueous is trapped in the posterior chamber of the eye between the iris and lens. Making a hole in the iris (*iridectomy* or *iridotomy*) allows aqueous to flow freely into the anterior chamber so deepening it and widening the drainage angle.

In *chronic glaucoma*, when the drainage of aqueous through the trabecular meshwork is impaired, a drainage operation may be necessary. A fistula is created which allows the aqueous to drain through the sclera into the subconjunctival space. The most commonly employed operation is a *trabeculectomy*. A trap-door of sclera, hinged at the corneoscleral junction, is raised and a block of trabecular tissue is excised.

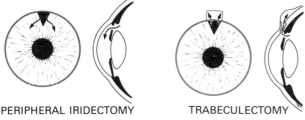

PERIPHERAL IRIDECTOMY   TRABECULECTOMY

Trabeculectomy drainage bleb.

Lasers are used in the treatment of glaucoma to produce *iridotomies* and also to improve the outflow of aqueous through the trabecular meshwork (*laser trabeculoplasty*). This is achieved by producing a series of minute scars which stretch the trabecular meshwork and open the spaces.

Dacryocystorhinostomy (DCR)

The purpose of this operation is to establish free drainage of tears into the nose. A fistula is created by anastomosing the mucosa of the lacrimal sac to that of the nasal cavity following removal of the intervening bone with a trephine or bone punch.

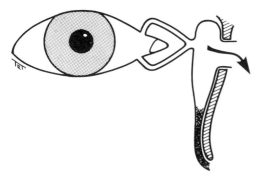

Surgical procedures

Cryotherapy

The sudden expansion of gas produces a lowering of temperature. Modern cryosurgical instruments use carbon dioxide or nitrous oxide. The main ophthalmic uses are:

1. CATARACT SURGERY

The probe adheres to the lens by the formation of an iceball. This is used to assist in the removal of the lens (intracapsular method).

2. RETINAL SURGERY

The probe is placed on the sclera to produce an iceball which encompasses the underlying retina and choroid. This produces an inflammatory reaction (chorioretinitis) which results in a strong adhesion between these two structures. It is used to seal retinal tears.

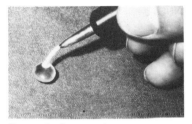
Cryoprobe frozen to lens.

3. TRICHIASIS

Repeated freezing of the lid margin is used to permanently remove ingrowing lashes without damaging the lid tissues.

4. GLAUCOMA

The secretory epithelium of the ciliary processes can be damaged by repeated freezing through the sclera. The rate of aqueous formation is reduced, leading to lower intraocular pressure though this is an uncertain method of treating the disease.

Photocoagulation

The *xenon arc* photocoagulator produces intense white light which is focused to produce a burn on the retina.

Laser light, particularly the continuous green light from the argon laser, produces burns of a more discreet size and has largely superseded the xenon arc photocoagulator.

Laser photocoagulation is used in the treatment of:

1. *Diabetic retinopathy*.
2. *Macular degeneration* (if subretinal neovascularization present).
3. Sealing *retinal holes and tears*. It cannot, however, be used when the retina is detached; chorioretinal apposition must be present.
4. *Iridotomy and trabeculoplasty*.

Newer lasers are now used in ophthalmology such as the YAG, which, with its very high energy output, allows intraocular membranes to be cut without resorting to invasive surgery.

Ocular pharmacology 36

A wide range of drugs is used in ocular therapy. Many of these have local and systemic side effects which must be appreciated by the doctor and explained to the patient. Conversely, drugs used in the treatment of systemic disorders may have serious ocular side effects including loss of vision.

Ocular therapy

The following drugs are commonly used in the diagnosis and treatment of eye disorders.

Adrenergic drugs

Adrenaline (Epinephrine)

This is used as a 0.5–2% solution in the treatment of open angle glaucoma. The outflow of aqueous from the eye is increased. *Side effects* are conjunctival hyperaemia and pigmentation and tachycardia. Acute angle closure glaucoma may be precipitated in eyes with narrow angles.

Phenylephrine

Used as a 5–10% solution to dilate the pupil for diagnostic purposes. It acts on the sympathetically innervated dilator pupillae muscle. *Side effects* are uncommon. Acute glaucoma may be precipitated and systemic hypertension has been reported.

Guanethidine

Used as a 1–3% solution in conjunction with adrenaline in the treatment of open angle glaucoma.

Side effects are conjunctival hyperaemia and a pharmacological Horner's syndrome (ptosis and miosis) resulting from sympathetic denervation.

Timolol

This beta-blocker is used as a 0.25–0.5% solution in the treatment of chronic glaucoma. It lowers the intraocular pressure by reducing the rate of aqueous formation. *Side effects* are the result of systemic absorption and include asthma and bradycardia. Ocular side effects are uncommon.

Parasympathetic drugs

Atropine   - Anticholinergics

This is used as a 1% solution or ointment for both diagnostic and therapeutic purposes. It acts as a mydriatic by paralysing the sphincter pupillae and as a cycloplegic by paralysing the ciliary muscle and abolishing accommodation. It is a long acting drug, the effects lasting up to 10 days. Similar but shorter acting drugs include *homatropine* (1–2%) which lasts for 2–3 days, *cyclopentolate* (0.5–1%) and *tropicamide* (0.5–1%) both of which last for a few hours. *Side effects* include blurred vision, particularly for close work, and dazzle. There is a small risk of precipitating acute glaucoma in eyes with narrow angles.

Pilocarpine

This cholinergic drug is widely used as a 1–4% solution in the treatment of glaucoma. In chronic glaucoma it increases the outflow of aqueous humour through the trabecular meshwork by causing contraction of the ciliary muscle. The pupil-constricting effect of pilocarpine is used in the treatment of acute glaucoma. *Side effects* include dimming of vision (due to miosis), myopia in the young (due to contraction of the ciliary muscle) and transient headache.

Phospholine iodide

An anticholinesterase, this drug is occasionally used as a 0.06–0.25% solution in the treatment of chronic glaucoma and accommodative squint. Its actions are similar to pilocarpine but it is longer acting. *Side effects* include cataract and iris cyst formation. Prolonged apnoea may occur if succinylcholine is used during general anaesthesia of a patient treated with phospholine iodide because levels of pseudo-cholinesterase, which normally rapidly destroy the muscle relaxant, are reduced.

Local antibiotics

Chloramphenicol

A broad-spectrum antibiotic that is widely used as a 0.5% solution or ointment in the treatment of bacterial infections of the anterior segment of the eye. *Side effects* are uncommon, even with prolonged usage though allergic reactions may occur.

Neomycin

Frequently used in combination with corticosteroids in proprietary preparations. Contact dermatitis is the most frequent *side effect* of this drug.

Gentamicin

This is effective against gram-negative bacterial infections of the eye including pseudomonas and proteus. *Side effects* include damage to the corneal epithelium following prolonged usage.

Antiviral Agents

Idoxuridine (IDU)

An antimetabolite, this drug is effective in the treatment of herpes simplex keratitis. It is used as a 0.1% solution every hour or as a 0.5% ointment five times daily. Other local antiviral agents include *vidarabine* and *acyclovir*. These are available as 3% ointments. *Side effects* include temporary damage to the corneal epithelium and blockage of the lacrimal puncta with prolonged use.

Local steroids

A wide spectrum of local steroid drops and ointments is available. In increasing order of potency these include hydrocortisone, prednisolone, betamethasone and dexamethasone. They are used in a wide variety of inflammatory disorders of the anterior segment of the eye. They are ineffective in treating inflammation of the optic nerve, retina or choroid and systemic steroids must be given when required. *Side effects* include the potentiation of herpes simplex virus and other microbial and fungal infections. In susceptible individuals glaucoma may be caused. Newer topical steroids such as fluoromethalone and clobetasone are said to be safer in this last respect.

Topical anaesthetic agents

Cocaine is rarely used these days as an ocular anaesthetic agent. Synthetic derivatives such as amethocaine and benoxinate are rapid in action and of relatively short duration. *Side effects* include serious corneal damage if the cornea is repeatedly anaesthetized over a long period of time. For this reason anaesthetic drops should not be prescribed for patients with painful corneal conditions.

Carbonic anhydrase inhibitors

Acetazolamide

This drug is taken orally in a dose of 125–250 mg every 6 hours for the treatment of chronic glaucoma. It is also given intramuscularly or intravenously in acute glaucoma. It acts by reducing the formation of aqueous humour. *Side effects* are common and include paraesthesiae of the extremities (in nearly all patients), depression, lethargy, indigestion and renal stone formation.

Dichlorphenamide

May be used as an alternative to acetazolamide but the side effects are similar.

Ocular toxicology

The following drugs, commonly used in the treatment of systemic diseases, may cause ocular side effects.

Corticosteroids

If used in doses of greater than 10 mg prednisolone per day (or equivalent) for periods of longer than a year there is a significant risk of *cataract* formation. These are characteristically of the posterior subcapsular type.

Ethambutol

Used in the treatment of tuberculosis, this drug may cause visual loss through either *optic nerve or retinal damage*.

Chloroquine

This drug, used in treatment of rheumatoid arthritis and systemic lupus erythematosus, accumulates in the body and may cause severe visual loss by damaging the *macula*. Corneal deposits of the drug are common but relatively harmless.

Sulphonamides

This is the most commonly incriminated group of drugs in the causation of the *Stevens–Johnson syndrome* (*see* Chapter 31).

Practolol

This systemic beta-blocker (now withdrawn) was responsible for many cases of severe *corneal and conjunctival scarring*. Other systemic beta-blockers appear to be safe in this respect.

Amiodarone

Used in the treatment of cardiac arrhythmias. *Corneal deposits* are frequently seen but are of no serious significance. They may cause slight reduction of vision and halo formation but the deposits disappear on discontinuation of the drug.

Digitalis

In high (or over-) dosage an alteration in colour vision may be appreciated by the patient. Objects take on a yellow hue.

Chlorpromazine

This drug, used in very high doses in the treatment of psychiatric disorders, may cause *pigmentation of the cornea and retina*.

Anticholinergic drugs

Many of these drugs, used as antidepressants or in the treatment of Parkinson's disease, may theoretically cause dilatation of the pupil with the risk of precipitating acute glaucoma. Although this can occur the risk is very small.

Common misconceptions

37

There are as many, if not more, misconceptions (or 'old wives' tales') about the eyes as any other part of the body. These may be a cause of concern to patients or even lead to inappropriate investigation and treatment.

1. The eyes are not damaged by:

a. Reading in poor light.
b. Sitting too close to a television.
c. Excessive use (for example reading, sewing or typing).
d. Using spectacles with the incorrect prescription (with rare exceptions in childhood).

2. Myopia does not reverse in middle age. However, the good near vision associated with this condition means that reading glasses (for presbyopia) are often not required.

3. A person with only one eye is no more likely to lose the vision in that eye than if he had two functioning eyes; it cannot be 'strained' by use.

4. Children do not grow out of a squint. Any child who appears to have a squint should be examined by an ophthalmologist as soon as possible.

5. The regular use of eye lotions, eyewashes and eye baths has no beneficial effect on the eyes.

6. A healthy person eating a normal diet does not require supplementary vitamins for the benefit of his eyes.

7. Eye 'exercises' can not reverse myopia or delay the need for reading glasses. Orthoptic exercises are designed to improve binocular function.

8. 'Spots' in front of the eyes have a local cause such as vitreous degeneration and are not a reflection of general ill-health or a sign of liver disease.

9. Migraine is not caused by refractive error or imbalance of the extraocular muscles.

10. The eye is not removed from the socket and laid on the cheek for surgery!

Index